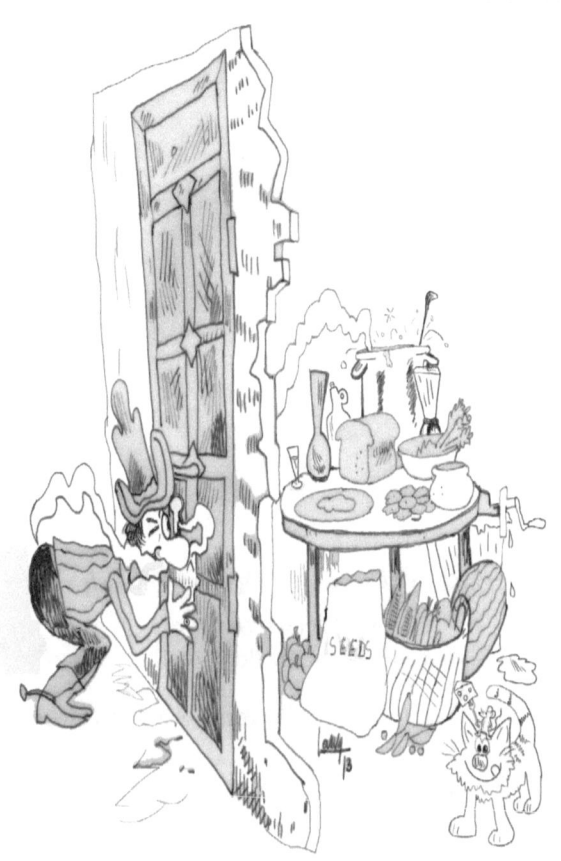

Hempseed Food:
the REAL Secret Ingredient for Health & Happiness

by Mariann Garner-Wizard

A Dharma Wizard Book
www.WordsWorth.biz
Austintatious, Aztlán/Austin, TX

Cover and chapter head drawings by Charlie Loving.
See more of his work at http://p-a-wood.com/CharlesLoving

ISBN: 978-1-304-51601-5
Printed in the United States of America.

And G-d said, "Behold, I have given you every plant yielding seed that is on the face of the earth, and every tree with seed in its fruit; you shall have them for food."
— Genesis 1:29, *Holy Bible,* Revised Standard Edition

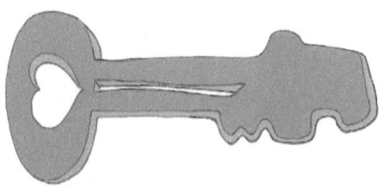

"And as I looked and wept, I saw that there stood on the north side of the starving camp a sacred man, who was painted all over his body, and he held a spear as he walked into the center of the people, and there he lay down and rolled. And when he got up, it was a fat bison standing there, and where the bison stood a sacred herb sprang up... The herb... bore four blossoms on a single stem while I was looking... and the bright rays of them flashed to the heavens.

"I now know what this meant: that the bison were the gift of a good spirit and were our strength, but we lost them, and from the same good spirit we must find another strength."
— **Black Elk**, medicine man and warrior of the Oglala Sioux

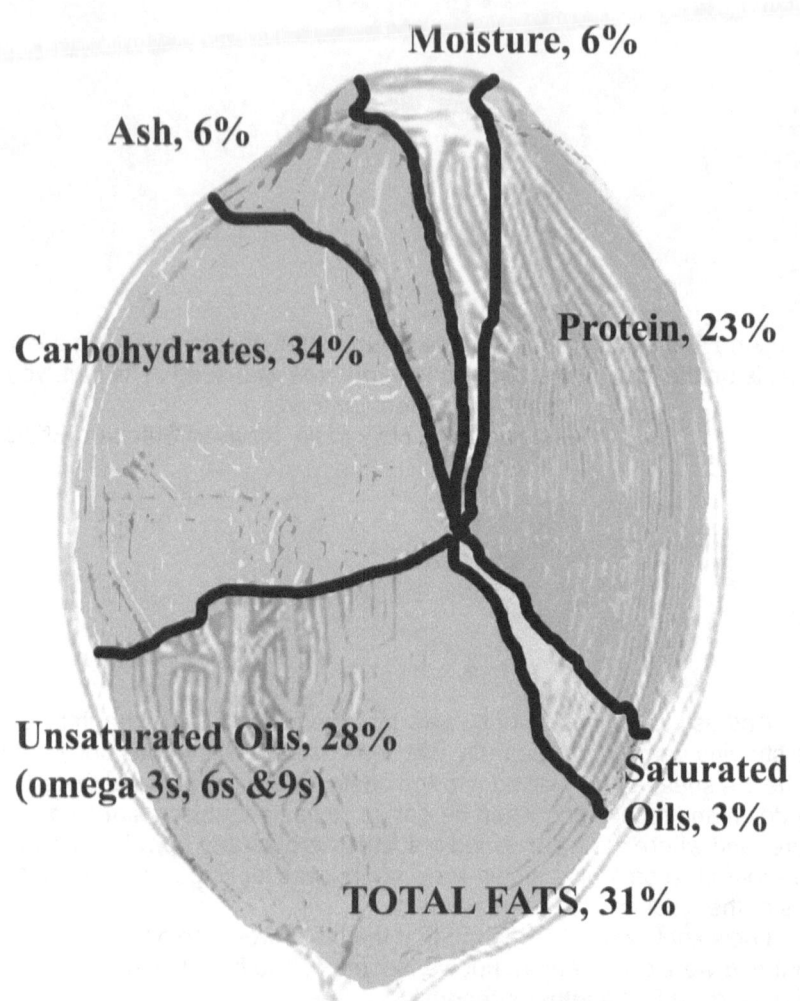

Moisture, 6%

Ash, 6%

Carbohydrates, 34%

Protein, 23%

Unsaturated Oils, 28%
(omega 3s, 6s &9s)

Saturated
Oils, 3%

TOTAL FATS, 31%

Inside the Hempseed:
Basic Nutritional Content

Figure 1.

Acknowledgments

This book has taken many years to reach fruition. Some recipes herein were created for *Don't Tread on Me*, a weekly live pro-Hemp television program produced by Hardware & Images and cablecast on Austin, Texas' public access Channel 10, then-managed by Austin Community Television, in 1993-1994 (see www.ChannelAustin.org).

I am grateful to the Hempseed cooks who inspired me: **Judy & Lynn Osburn, Carol Miller & Don Wirtshafter, Mary Rathbun & Dennis Peron**, and **Tom Flowers**. Great steps in Hempseed nutrition have come from the mind, energy, and enterprise of **Richard Rose**, father of today's Hemp food industry. Many internet sites now feature Hempseed foods.

I salute those who kept alive through perilous times the knowledge that Cannabis itself is edible and delicious: **Chef Ra**, *High Times* magazine; **Evelyn Schmevelyn; Conrad J Camille**; the unknown author(s) of *Supermother's Cooking With Grass*, and the foxy lady who first hipped me to it, **Ita Jones**. The *Medical Marijuana Handbook* gave early recipes for "medical edibles."

Udo Erasmus' *Fats and Oils* remains the definitive work on the role of fats and oils in nutrition and health.

Jack Herer, Freedom Fighter #1, author of *The Emperor Wears No Clothes*, opened my mind to the fact that Hemp was good for something besides my head. One Love to Bro. Jack of blessed memory, and all the **Freedom Fighters** still doing their part!

In writing this book, I benefited from the knowledge of many cannabis activists. **Allen St. Pierre**, Director, National Organization for the Reform of Marijuana Laws (NORML); Brazilian researcher **AW Zuardi**; California NORML director and vaporizer co-inventor **Dale Gieringer**; and **Jon Gettman**, Editor, *Bulletin of Cannabis Reform*, all responded generously to my occasional queries. *Mis amigos* **Kate & John, Liz & Frank**, and **Sally & David** shared their enthusiasm and culinary expertise. Last but not least, **Vicki** and **Beverly** each found my typos and other errors.

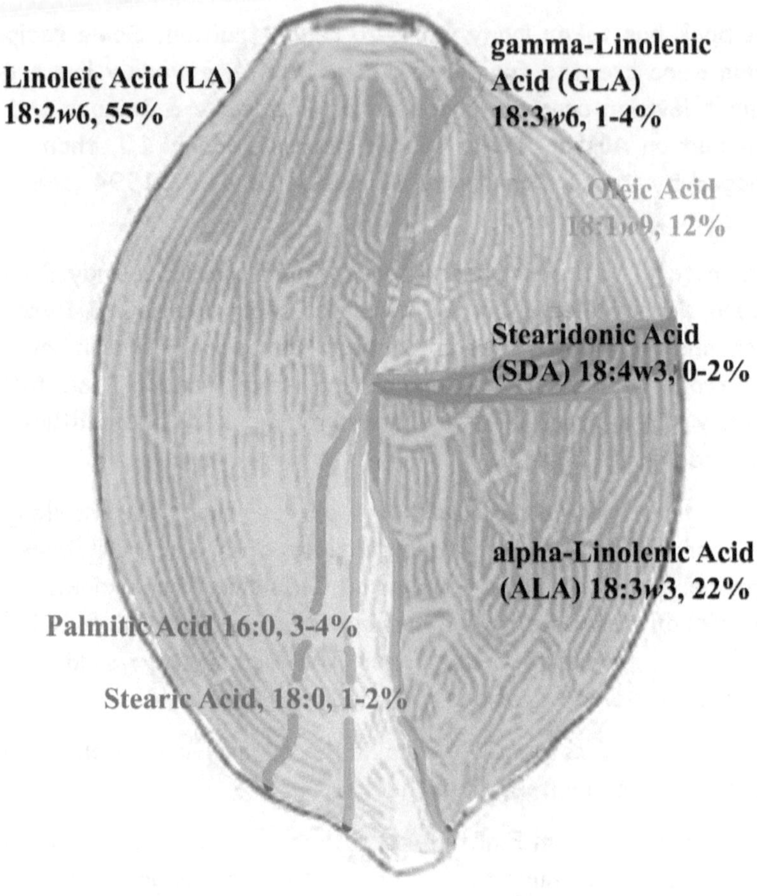

Linoleic Acid (LA)
18:2*w*6, 55%

gamma-Linolenic
Acid (GLA)
18:3*w*6, 1-4%

Oleic Acid
18:1*w*9, 12%

Stearidonic Acid
(SDA) 18:4w3, 0-2%

alpha-Linolenic Acid
(ALA) 18:3*w*3, 22%

Palmitic Acid 16:0, 3-4%

Stearic Acid, 18:0, 1-2%

Inside the Hempseed:
Fatty Acid Content

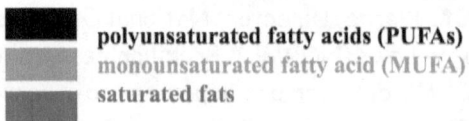

■ **polyunsaturated fatty acids (PUFAs)**
■ monounsaturated fatty acid (MUFA)
■ saturated fats

Figure 2

Dedications

With appreciation to **J Lynn Lively-Beauman** & **Cassie Vizard**, who shanghaied me into being their video hempseed cook; **Michael L Kleinman, Matthew M Kleinman-Wizard, Roland D DeNoie,** & **W Andrew Beauman,** who ate it all up; **Mark Hanel, Richard Douglas** (both of blessed memory), & **David Martinez** for the perfect Cannabis Test Kitchen; & the volunteer cast & crew of *Don't Tread on Me*, especially producer **Josephine D Mays.**

With growing hope to companions in the struggle: **Cathy & Arlin "US Hemp" Troutt & Family** in AZ; **Lennie Moren, Linda Ronan,** & **Tim Hinterberger** in Anchorage and **Dirk Nelson** in Ester, AK; the **Thiede Family** in CO; **Jonah Raskin,** the **Goddesses of Mendocino, Mary M, Bob'n'Helen, AverLou,** the other **Mark Kleiman,** & friends too numerous to name in CA; & the **Texas Hemp Campaign, Texas NORML Women's Alliance,** Mayor of Houston's Fift' Ward **Robert "Bob" Al-Walee,** & **Howard & Karen Wooldridge** and **"Misty"** of **Citizens Opposing Prohibition** (COP) among hundreds of fellow Texans around the world.

With love to my strongest and wisest allies. San Marcos community lodestar, dance diva, artist, videographer, and exemplary mother **Vicki Hartin** has supported this and other projects dear to my heart with unstinting skill, laughter, and devotion. **Mark Blumenthal,** Founder and Executive Director of the **American Botanical Council** (www.herbalgram.org) has helped me hone my knowledge of cannabis medicine, regulatory policy, and nutrition by inviting me to write for ABC's peer-reviewed publications. My son **Matt** not only tried many test recipes but is a constant inspiration and strength in my life. He also contributed the **Hempseed Milk Curry Sauce** recipe on p. 46! Without their encouragement and urging, this book would remain an unsprouted seed.

And *with pleasure* to the other **Richard Lee** in the Zombie Motor City.

One Love!
mgw, 30 September 2013

Recipe Notes

Contents

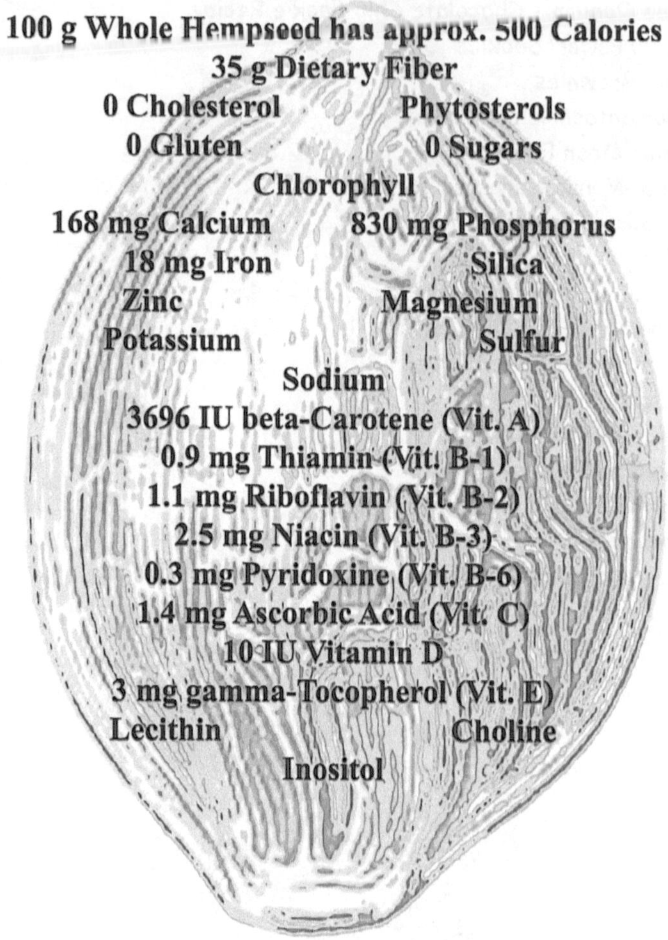

100 g Whole Hempseed has approx. 500 Calories
35 g Dietary Fiber
0 Cholesterol   Phytosterols
0 Gluten   0 Sugars
Chlorophyll
168 mg Calcium   830 mg Phosphorus
18 mg Iron   Silica
Zinc   Magnesium
Potassium   Sulfur
Sodium
3696 IU beta-Carotene (Vit. A)
0.9 mg Thiamin (Vit. B-1)
1.1 mg Riboflavin (Vit. B-2)
2.5 mg Niacin (Vit. B-3)
0.3 mg Pyridoxine (Vit. B-6)
1.4 mg Ascorbic Acid (Vit. C)
10 IU Vitamin D
3 mg gamma-Tocopherol (Vit. E)
Lecithin   Choline
Inositol

Inside the Hempseed:
Vitamins, Minerals & Other Nutrients

Contents may vary with genetic characteristics, growth environment,
and maturity at harvest. Amounts shown are representative.
An average serving might include 20 g Hempseed.

Figure 3

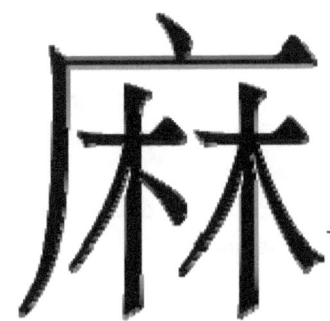

Chinese Ideogram "Ma"

Two hemp plants hang under a drying hut roof.

It is said that the Buddha once lived
for six years by eating
just one Hempseed a day.

Preface

In what is now northwest China 10-15,000 years ago, humans first began to plant seeds. Along with millet and rice, a tall leafy plant called *ma* (above) was one of the first foods cultivated. Its seeds, rich in energy, were also an early fuel source. The same plant was the first crop grown for textile fiber. Its stalks give the strongest natural fibers known. Cloth made from the outer fiber has been dated as over 9000 years old. And long before it was planted anywhere, the plant grew wild, and likely was used for ropes, nets, and snares. When paper-making was invented, the fibrous stalks had yet another use.

Ma has names in every language; in most, several. Many are variations on Greek *kanabis*, itself probably from ancient Assyrian *quunubu* or *qunupu*, one of the oldest words surviving in modern times. Many Afro-Eurasian texts, from Egyptian papyrus scrolls to Mesopotamian clay tablets, discuss medical uses of this plant as though it had been in use long before they were written. Assyrian medical texts 4000 years old give no sign that its uses were recent discoveries. Greek and Roman texts mention experiments to find new uses for what was by then a very familiar medicine.

Leonhard Fuchs gave the plant its now-standard Latin name, *Cannabis sativa*, "useful cannabis," in 1542 CE.[1] In English it was "cannabis hemp" (from German *hanf*) from early Anglo-Saxon times until the 1920s, when certain competing interests in the United

xiii

---

[1] Russo E. History of *Cannabis* and its preparations in saga, science, and sobriquet. *Chemistry & Biodiversity*. 2007;4:1614-1648.

States began to call it by a Mexican slang term; *marihuana*. We call it cannabis, or hemp, or marijuana.

For thousands of years hempseed was an important food for nutrition and good health not only in China, but from India to Siberia and west to England. It crossed the Atlantic Ocean with early explorers and "New World" settlers of every nationality and status, but had been known in the West from time immemorial.[2]

In the 1920s, 30s, and 40s, anti-"*marihuana*" campaigns virtually erased hempseed's culinary uses from popular culture, history, and knowledge, and from the world's tables. Hempseed and other "old-fashioned" whole foods were bypassed for bleached flour, refined sugar, "stabilized" oil, and other foods made commercially rather than locally or at home.

Today, new research, especially in Israel, Spain, Brazil, and Great Britain, is finding new medical uses for cannabis' unique compounds, including those in hempseed. Hempseed's linoleic acid content has anti-inflammatory properties. Hemp oil relieves atopic dermatitis (eczema).[3] Hempseed and hempseed oil have shown benefits in multiple sclerosis patients.[4]

Use of environmentally friendly hemp fiber for textiles, paper, and even construction materials and auto parts is rising. Hemp's

---

[2] Craker LE, Gardner Z. The botany of Cannabis. **The Pot Book**, ed. Holland J. Park Street Press, Toronto. 2010. Unfortunately, what was known by Native Americans before Europeans found the Western Hemisphere is unclear today. It seems unlikely that there was a strong tradition of medicinal use, however, due to a prehistoric division of the Cannabis plant into two major types: one best at producing strong fibers; the other best at producing resinous flowers. Although the varieties interbreed with ease, the fibrous variety was prevalent in the New World. In addition, many indigenous herbal medicines are still used traditionally; some are known from the work of Eclectic physicians who learned from Native Americans. But cannabis wasn't added to their "patent medicines" until after the more resinous variety was introduced to Europe, and thence the Americas, from the Far East.

[3] Callaway JC, Schwab U, Harvimaa I, et. al. Efficacy of dietary hempseed oil in patients with atopic dermatitis. *Journal of Dermatological Treatment*. 2005;16:87-94.

[4] Rezapour-Firouzi S, Arefhosseini SR, Farhoudi M, et. al. Association of Expanded Disability Status Scale and cytokines after intervention with co-supplemented hemp seed, evening primrose oils and hot-natured diet in multiple sclerosis patients. *Biolimpacts*. 2013;3(1):43-47. Available at: http://www.ncbi.nlm.nih.gov/pmc/articles/PMC3648912.

cellulose content is a potential source of ethanol; spent fiber is a potential source of biomass fuel. Hundreds of hemp-based products, from soaps, shampoos, and other personal care items to crafters' supplies enjoy robust sales in the US – using hemp grown in Canada, China, and 30 or more other agricultural nations.

Worldwide, prohibitions against "useful cannabis" are falling. In the US 20 states have voted to allow some cultivation of fibrous hemp, but farmers cannot yet grow it due to opposition from the federal Drug Enforcement Administration (DEA).[5]

Hempseed foods have come back too, defeating US government opposition, and are available at most health food stores and some mainstream grocers. However, most are to some degree processed. *It's as if we had canned corn, corn oil, corn syrup, cornstarch, and corn muffins, but no corn on the cob!*

Today the developed world, including the US, is experiencing a health crisis. Diabetes, cancer, heart disease, and other chronic illnesses are increasing. "One out of two Americans will die from... cardiovascular disease (CVD). One out of four... will die from cancer... Pioneers in... biochemistry and human nutrition now believe CVD and most cancers are... caused by... over-consumption of saturated fats and refined vegetable oils that turn *essential fatty acids* (EFAs) into carcinogenic killers... Ignorance of human nutritional needs... will cause [an] overwhelming majority... to die... from these afflictions - the greatest killers in affluent nations."[6]

Is it a coincidence that these chronic conditions began to increase sharply when fresh-pressed oils and whole grains, including those from hemp, disappeared from the typical Western diet?

Marketers often advertise "secret" or "new" ingredients to boost their products' appeal. While not at all new, hempseed has

---

[5] Johnson R. Hemp as an agricultural commodity. *Congressional Research Service.* March 21, 2013; RL32725.
[6] Osburn L. Hemp seed: the most nutritionally complete food source in the world. *Hemp Line Journal,* July-Aug. 1992; I(1):14-15. (*Italics added.*)

become a *real* "secret ingredient," its valuable protein and essential oils lost to most people and underused by the rest. **No more!**

I've selected a variety of recipes for **Hempseed Food**, showcasing the many traditions and techniques this versatile grain can enrich. Read on to learn more about the benefits of using *real, natural hempseed!*

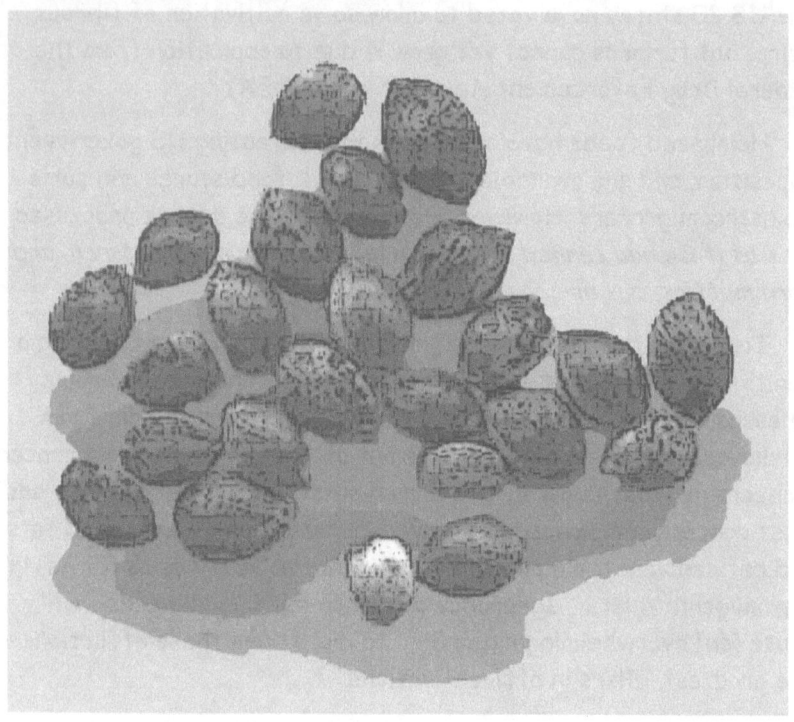

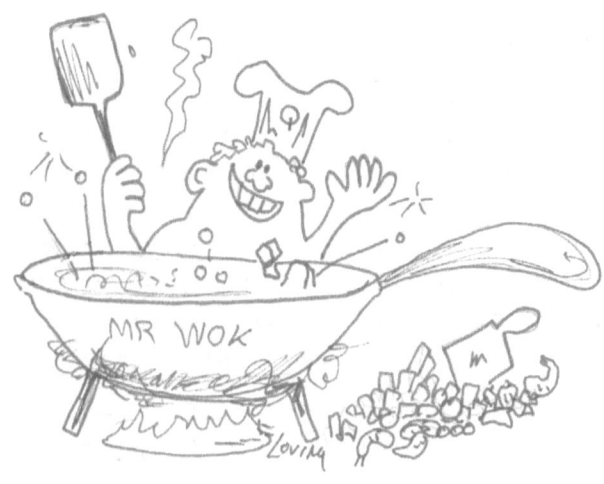

Hempseed: a Functional Food

"Functional foods" have potentially positive effects on health beyond basic nutrition. Without doubt, hempseed is a valuable functional food.

Hempseed is the fruit of cannabis, a plant that produces fiber for rope, canvas, fabric, carpets, and paper in an endlessly renewable supply; oil and biomass for fuel; and whose leaves and flowers, if smoked or eaten, produce feelings of euphoria and clarity, sometimes referred to as "being high."

Hempseed, however, doesn't alter the consciousness. It is simply the most nutritious food known to humanity, enjoyed for centuries worldwide. In Dickens' *Oliver Twist*, when Oliver asks, "Please, sir, may I have some more gruel?" he's asking for Hempseed porridge (see **Twisted Hempseed Gruel**, p. 58)! From soup to tasty desserts, Hempseed does it all!

Certain "good fats" contribute to good health. Fresh-pressed "live" oils used for cooking and flavor throughout history were driven from the market in recent decades by cooking oil companies seeking a stable shelf life. Hempseed returns fresh oils to our diet. Just two edible oils (from flaxseed and Hempseed) have significant amounts of EFAs: lin-o-lé-ic (LA; omega-6) and alpha lin-o-lén-ic (ALA; omega-

3), both vital for human life. Hempseed has more LA (21%) and less ALA (7%) than flaxseed (5% LA; 20% ALA). It is about 30-35% oil by weight (**Figs. 1** and **2**). Of all edible oils, only Hempseed has omega-3s, omega-6s, and gamma-linoleic acid (GLA; omega-9). Unlike flaxseed, Hempseed oil can be used continuously without EFA imbalances or deficiencies. Polyunsaturated fatty acids (PUFAs) and phytosterols, found in high amounts in Hempseed, lower risks of heart disease; phytosterols by lowering cholesterol. Hempseed foods legally make regulated "heart healthy" claims in the US. Phytosterols and chlorophyll both add to its anti-cancer component.

Whole Hempseeds have 23% protein (**Fig. 1**) and 17 amino acids, including all 10 *essential amino acids* (EAAs). **That's more than beef!** They have cysteine and methionine, sulfur-bearing EAAs seldom found in plant foods. Hempseed protein is one-third globulin edestin and two-thirds albumins, similar to egg whites, and can be used raw by the body. (Soybeans must be cooked or sprouted for digestion.) Hempseed's 1:2 edestin-albumin ratio may echo prehistoric diets. Its protein is especially valuable for vegetarians and vegans.

Hempseed has vitamins A, C, B-1, B-2, B-3, B-6, D, & E; the nutrients lecithin, choline, & inositol; and minerals potassium, calcium, magnesium, phosphorus, silica, iron, sulfur, & zinc. Hulls are 35% insoluble dietary fiber. Hempseed has no cholesterol.

Can something so healthy still taste good? Yes! Even "junk food junkies" love the rich, nutty taste! But don't worry, hempseeds are *not* nuts, and people allergic to nuts, wheat, soy, and gluten can safely eat them! A low glycemic index, about 35% carbohydrates, and nutrients that help control blood sugar, makes them safe for diabetics as well. Hempseed milk is lactose free. Hempseed has about 500 calories per 100 grams, but few recipes in this book call for as much as 20 grams per serving.

Why is Hempseed a "Secret Ingredient"?

So, if Hempseed is so good, why don't we all eat it? Why is it such a secret? To answer this fully would take a social and political history of the past century, well beyond my humble aims! There are many sources for this information (see *Links & Resources*).

But, hemp was vitally important when the United States was founded. Sailing ships carrying settlers to the New World each used, with their equipment and sailors' clothes and shoes, 30+ tons of Hemp and its products; "Old Ironsides" used 60 tons. Hemp fabric, called "homespun" because every home made it, clothed most settlers. Hemp paper was cheap, acid-free, and sturdy; if books were scarce, they were long-lasting. And Hempseed "grits" and "gruel" were nutritious foods for a growing country. The Founding Fathers knew Hemp was vital to national security and prosperity, America's "moral fiber."

But Hemp competed with some new, developing industries and some old, aristocratic attitudes. In post-Civil War days, when Black people began holding their heads higher than "Jim Crow" liked, smoking Hemp flowers and leaves ("gage"; "reefer") was linked with an "uppity" attitude. Women demanding their rights, especially sexual freedom, were seen as possible "drug addicts." Some Hispanics along the rapidly changing Western US border also used what Mexican rebel leader Pancho Villa called *marihuana*, and some in the US had begun to call "killer weed." Cultural and class conflict would continue to define cannabis' history in the US for 150 years.

An alliance between timber/pulp paper/newspaper baron William Randolph Hearst; the DuPont company, whose Nylon® petrochemical fabric had just been patented; and distillers recovering from Alcohol Prohibition came together in what would today be called *restraint of trade*, linking *marihuana* with undesirable social elements (people of color) and a decline in morals (sexual activity and sassing their elders) among youth. Tobacco and cotton farmers and the new synthetic drug industry also jumped on the anti-"dope" bandwagon.

The first local ordinance against marijuana was passed in 1914 in El Paso, TX, after a fight said to have been started by "a Mexican." By 1937 marijuana was illegal throughout the US, to the surprise of Hemp growers and the American Medical Association, who learned too late that the now-forbidden killer weed was none other than Cannabis Hemp!

Since then a "war on drugs" waged by the US government has sought not only to eradicate this useful plant but all knowledge of it. References to Hemp's once-central place in the economy were methodically scrubbed from textbooks, reference works, and libraries to protect its competitors.

According to NORML, nearly 8 million Americans were arrested for marijuana-related crimes between 2000-2010[7] alone, mostly for having ("possessing") some cannabis. The number rises yearly. A vast "prison industry" – a phrase that should be obscene! – profits from these arrests. The drug war has also been used as a battering ram against once-sacred civil liberties and the Bill of Rights.

Among the casualties of the war on drugs was Hempseed nutrition. But there was a loophole in anti-Hemp legislation: *exotic bird fanciers convinced Congress in 1937 that many birds needed Hempseed to sing*. Thus, sterilized Hempseed is legally imported for birdseed. It is largely due to this fact, and human curiosity, that the knowledge that Hempseed is both edible and delicious has survived!

This book revives the possibilities of Hempseed foods for everyday cooks. As with any "new" food, the creative cook will adapt these recipes to his or her style, availability of fresh produce, preference in spices, etc. A good cook's imagination, properly stimulated, gives rise to transient masterpieces of taste, texture, color, and aroma. Enjoy good meals in good company, enjoy good health, and "live good"[8] with Hempseed!

---

[7] —. Marijuana prosecutions for 2010 near record high. Sept. 19, 2011. http://norml.org/news/2011/09/19/marijuana-prosecutions-for-2010-near-record-high.

[8] With a tip of the hat, and fond remembrances of Roland Ord DeNoie, Esq., and Salvation Sandwiches.

* * STOP THE PRESSES!! A Policy Change? * *

Just as this book was being finalized, news broke that the US may have turned a corner in the war on drugs and might be ready to call a truce. On August 29, 2013, US Attorney General Eric Holder announced that the federal government would not seek to overturn citizen-initiated laws allowing recreational cannabis use in Colorado and Washington states, or state laws allowing medical marijuana use. This may even help clear the way for industrial or food-grade hemp agriculture and production! Lower prices for hempseed foods and other hemp products, along with jobs and economic growth, could follow such decisions.

While this announced shift in federal policy comes with several caveats and lacks the force of law, by removing immediate threats of federal intervention from states' decision-making processes, it negates a once-powerful argument against pro-cannabis initiatives and legislation: "*It doesn't matter what we do, the federal government can just overturn it.*" While still technically the case, a window has been opened for states to enact responsible, fair legislation to gain the benefits of cannabis' many attributes.

Notes on "Marijuana"

Though Hempseed can't alter consciousness, if that is your goal, many people find that medicinal and spiritual effects of "marijuana" (cannabis flowers and leaves) are better obtained through digestion than inhalation. Fresh, raw marijuana may be added to almost any food. Its texture and appearance are improved by grinding or chopping before use.

Because marijuana's psychoactive compounds aren't water- but fat-soluble, the most unobtrusive and efficient way to cook with it is in butter. Such herbed butter is not to be confused with **Hempseed butter** (page 12). Here are two ways to make "electric butter," one with a variation:

5

1. Gently sauté an ounce of herb in 4 oz. (one stick) of dairy butter until butter turns about the same color as the herb used. Strain out and discard plant material. Cool, cover, and refrigerate butter until hard, or use while still melted, in recipes or at the table.

2. a) Cover 6 cups fresh leaves in water and barely simmer for an hour or longer. Add 8 oz. (two sticks) dairy butter; simmer for another hour. Strain leaf fiber out, press, set liquid aside, and return fiber to the pot. Pour more boiling water over the fiber. When it cools press as much liquid from it as possible, adding liquid to that from the first pressing. Repeat. Discard fiber. Refrigerate liquid overnight. Skim the green butter off and refrigerate, covered, until use.

b) Cover 1 oz. fresh leaves and 1 lb. (4 sticks) of butter well with water. Heat just to a simmer. Turn off heat; allow to cool. Repeat three times; chill overnight. Chilled butter is easy to remove from water and spent herb.

Cannabis should not be heated above the boiling point, 212° F. Delta-9-tetrahydrocannabinol (Δ^9-THC), its main psychoactive ingredient, and other cannabinoids vaporize at 185-190° F. Once extracted into fats they can be cooked at much higher temperatures without vaporizing. Cannabis butter may be substituted for dairy butter in any recipe in this book.

Medical cannabis dispensaries in many cities offer gourmet treats made with specially grown cannabis to qualified buyers. Most "medical edibles" so far tend toward chocolate and sweetness. The **Twice-Baked Idaho POTato** (p. 41) was inspired by this author's too-great indulgence in sugary stuff in San Francisco on a 2005 research trip. I've also included cannabis-containing recipes that don't rely on refined flour or sugar. In some adapted from yesteryear's "underground" marijuana cookbooks, the "electric" ingredient (⚡) is left in; however, you may omit it from any recipe herein with a loss, perhaps, only of appreciation!

Cannabis may also be extracted by soaking in olive or other high-quality seed oil for several days. Use in salad dressings and other cold-oil applications. Early Christians may have used such an extract to anoint themselves and as a topical medicine. Warm cannabis oil is sometimes used for earache. Heating cannabis in milk also extracts active compounds.

Some medical users and herbalists prefer tinctures, steeping cannabis in 80 proof ethanol alcohol for 48 hours. This is dispensed by the Tablespoonful, diluted.

Marijuana "tea" [9] - an infusion of cannabis flowers in very hot water - is highly regarded by some although THC is water-insoluble. When flowering tops are soaked in water, the resin-bearing glans wash off and are consumed, exerting relaxing, vasodilating effects.

* * *

Among the more insidious developments of the "war on drugs" - really a war on marijuana users - has been the rise of *urinalysis*. Workers, job-seekers, people on probation or parole, recipients of government assistance or benefits, and others regularly provide urine to be tested for THC metabolites. Trace amounts of THC in Hempseed foods, when a slight easing of the drug war gave us a brief taste of them in the 1970s, led the DEA to ban hemp foods for several years, until the courts overruled the ban. *One would have to eat a great deal of Hempseed to obtain a positive for THC on a urine test.* A Canadian laboratory analyzed six varieties of industrial Hempseed in 2000 and found THC levels from 0.40 parts per million (µg/g) to 4.66 µg/g, averaging 0.54–3.57 µg/g. [10] Most was on seed hulls, from contact with flowers and leaves; hulled Hempseed ("hempnut") had even less THC content.

* * *

Where people still rely for medical and recreational cannabis on Mexican imports, seeds make up much of the product, usually discarded by users. Hempseed's nutritional benefits and the chance to use these formerly unwanted nuggets, for which one may pay as much by weight as for "hempnut," may interest these consumers.

---

[9] There is only one true tea, *Camellia sinensis*. Other infusions or decoctions made with plant material and hot water are called "tea" for convenience and by popular convention.

[10] Hemp Oil Canada, Inc., Shaun Crew, President. Laboratory Analysis of THC Content in Industrial Hemp Seed. Mar. 10, 2000.

REMEMBER: Marijuana possession (including unsterilized seeds) remains illegal under US law. Cannabis is best used by adults, and must **never** be administered without consent. With those caveats, feel free to add "the Spice of Life" to any recipe in this book!

The Endocannabinoids and Hempseed Nutrition

Long after the drug war began, scientists found that we humans make our own cannabinoids ("endocannabinoids") and have cannabinoid receptors throughout our brains and bodies. This biological communication system, evolved over millennia, regulates brain chemicals affecting mood, sleep, appetite, memory, higher cognition, emotions, blood pressure, bone density, body temperature, fertility, metabolism, and more. Both endo- and exocannabinoids strongly protect nerves, the nervous system, and their operations.

All animals except insects have endocannabinoids and cannabinoid receptors.[11] Archaeology, history, language, and folk medicine show that humans have had a beneficial relationship with cannabis ever since our diets had the same proportion of proteins as Hempseed. Today, research is focused on identifying endocannabinoids, their functions, and receptor responses to exocannabinoids such as THC and cannabidiol (CBD, of great medical interest), other compounds in cannabis, and their metabolites.

This may be the first publication to link two fascinating facts:

1. Key endocannabinoids anandamide and 2-arachidonoyl glycerol (2-AG) are made by our bodies, as are other important signaling compounds, from arachidonic acid.[12]

2. Arachidonic acid, found in meat foods, is also made by the body from linoleic acid, found abundantly in hempseed.[13]

In other words, *nutrients in hempseed support the endocannabinoid system;* while *compounds in cannabis flowers can stimulate and regulate this same system.*

I believe this topic deserves serious exploration.

---

[11] Lee MA. **Smoke Signals**. Scribner, New York. 2012.
[12] Mechoulam R, Hanuš L. Anandamide and more. **The Pot Book**, *op. cit.*
[13] Erasmus U. **Fats and Oils**. Alive Books, Burnaby BC, Canada, 1986.

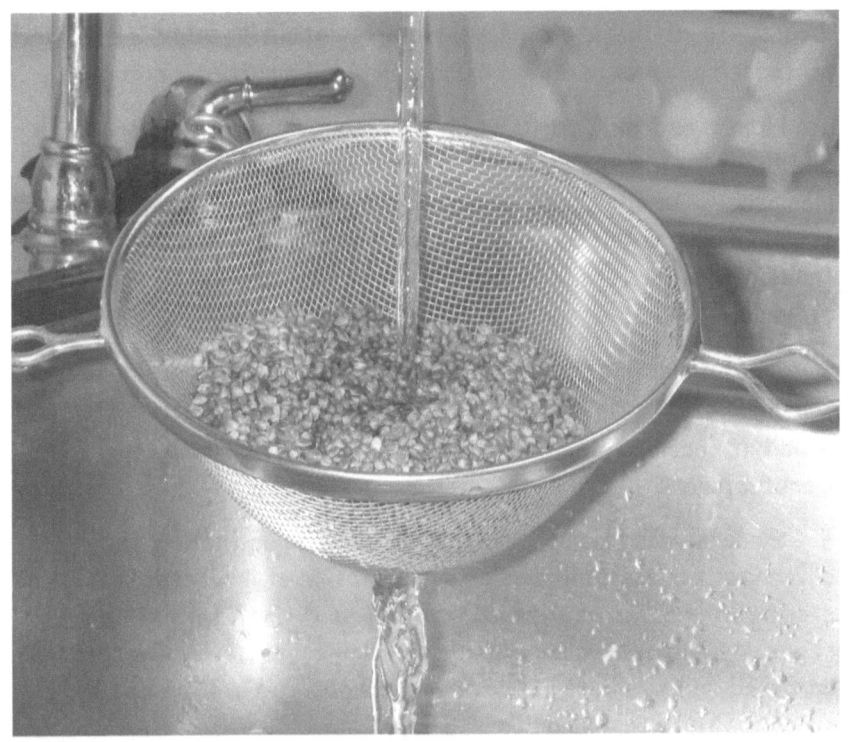

Hempseed Basics

Hempseed oil is available, although expensive, in health food and some mainstream groceries. Use Hempseed oil for salad dressings, fresh vegetable drizzles, marinades, and other foods using cold oil. Substitute it for olive oil in tabouley and hummus for a delightful taste. But *Do Not Cook With Hempseed Oil!* High heat destroys its food value and, as with other over-heated oils, creates "free radicals" the body can't readily digest.

Shelled or hulled Hempseed ("**hempnut**"; "hemp germ") is preferred over whole Hempseed by those who don't like crunchy foods or who value its convenience. Several cookbooks and websites offer hempnut recipes. However, hempnut has been much more expensive than whole Hempseed, yet lacks the vitamins and minerals in seed hulls. Also, consumers must check to see that hempnut products aren't made in facilities that process wheat, nuts, soy beans, etc., if this is a concern. **Hemp protein powder** is another processed product retaining much of whole hempseed's nutrition.

Hempseed milk, tofu or **cheese, yogurt**, and other products like those made from dairy milk or soybeans are made from Hempseeds. In China, special hemp strains produce huge seeds with abundant oil content for these foods. Hempseed milk is a lactose-free dairy substitute. You can find instructions online for making it at home.

Protein-rich **Hempseed cake**, produced when seeds are pressed for oil, is used in commercial Hemp foods and Hemp beer. Sifted and milled, it becomes **Hempseed flour**, also used by Hemp food manufacturers.

Since all living Hemp ("marijuana") is illegal in the US, the government doesn't allow sale or importation of live seed. It is steamed or heated at the port of entry so it won't sprout! This reduces nutritional value, but not by much.[14] (NOTE: If live seeds are sprouted, hulls fall off in two days. *Cannabis* sprouts can be used like sprouts of alfalfa, Mung beans, etc.)

---

[14] "[L]ittle damage is done to the seed by the steaming process... for a variety of reasons: 1) the coat is very hard and usually remains intact; 2) internal temperature of the seed is... well below 212° F; 3) the seed moves about as it is heated and thus can cool intermittently...; 4)... protein is not denatured by the process; 5) fats are not transformed at this temperature, although if a seed coat was broken it could begin to oxidize...; 6) birds continue to thrive on... sterilized seed; 7) the process was designed to apply the minimum amount of heat to render the seed nonviable while still maintaining nutrition for birds; and 8) most expeller-pressed hempseed oil is subjected to internal temperatures exceeding that of steaming, and for a longer period of time. However, I do believe that overall... degradation of "freshness" is accelerated by... sterilization..., most evident in seed stored for longer periods of time.

"The true senselessness of requiring sterilization of hempseed which is incapable of producing usable quantities of THC is that... sprouting... hempseed is the key to using it for many foods! Sprouting increases some nutrition, improves digestibility, reduces cost (one pound of seed will yield three pounds of sprouts...), and most importantly, improves ease of handling since the coats are split and can be removed with water agitation...

"This is why... countries that don't require sterilization have the edge in the production of hempseed foods..." – Richard Rose, Hempseed Foods. http://www.hempfood.com.

Some health food stores and mainstream groceries now carry **unshelled whole sterile hempseed**. It is also sold at feed and pet stores as birdseed. Canaries won't sing without it. Feed stores have historically had the best prices, but that may be changing as hempfoods' popularity soars. Whole hempseed can be found in bulk online. (See *Links & Resources*, p. 61.) But only when hempseed is grown domestically will prices stabilize!

A pound of seed makes about five cups of ground toasted Hempseed or raw ground Hempseed meal. Wash seeds well in running water.[15] Remove broken seeds. Seeds for birds may have been treated for pests, but not with poison — something bitter or hot is more likely; it will wash off. Most Hempseed in prepared foods and **hempnut** is certified organic.

Raw whole Hempseed   Toasted whole Hempseed

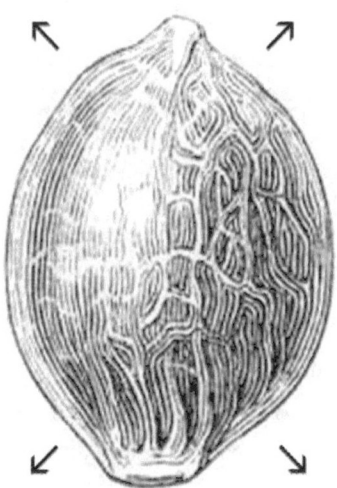

Raw ground Hempseed meal   Toasted ground Hempseed
+ Hempseed butter

Hempseed Basic Preparations

Figure 4.

---

[15] Compared with other agents, water removed surface THC from seeds more cost-effectively and worked as well. Hemp Oil Canada, Inc., Shaun Crew, President. Development of Hemp Food Products & Processes. Sept., 2000.

Enjoy **raw** or **toasted whole Hempseeds** plain or lightly salted. For basic Hempseed home cooking, there are two options: **raw ground Hempseed meal** or ground toasted Hempseed. **Raw ground Hempseed meal** is also the first step in making **Hempseed butter** (**NOT** cannabis butter). Most recipes in this book use these options. A few use **Hempseed oil, Hemp flour, hempnut,** or **Hempseed milk,** available at health food stores and finer grocers. Keep raw seeds frozen until needed. The sturdy hull protects the nutrients within!

1. For **raw ground Hempseed meal,** measure the quantity of seeds needed a few at a time into a spice or coffee grinder or food mill. Follow manufacturer's instructions. Grind until seeds are well broken-up; they are quite sticky due to the oil content. The finer you grind them, the less "gritty" they become. *For baking, especially, a fine grind is better.*

Baking with Hempseed Meal

Raw ground Hempseed meal may be substituted for 1/3 of the main dry ingredient and *all* of the shortening (fat or oil) in baking. If first results are too oily, reduce the amount of Hempseed; if too dry, increase it. (See **Breads & Pastries,** p. 49.)

1a. For **Hempseed butter,** strain **raw ground Hempseed** meal though a sifter, then grind what remains again. Mix the two grindings together , sift again, and repeat until you obtain a spread with the velvety consistency of peanut butter. Be patient, it's worth it!

2. A few recipes here use **whole toasted Hempseed**. Enjoy also in cereal, trail mix, or out-of-hand. Follow directions below for **ground toasted Hempseed** but skip the grinding.

2a. For **ground toasted Hempseed,** spread clean seeds – wet or dry – one layer deep on a cookie sheet and bake at 350° F for 4 minutes (dry) or just slightly longer (wet). Or toast small quantities in a covered skillet on the stove, shaking the pan gently and constantly for about 4 minutes at medium high heat. When you hear the seeds start to POP, remove from the heat! *Don't scorch your* *seeds!* You can toast seeds more darkly by using a lower temperature for a minute longer. Let seeds cool. Grind them a few at a time. Inhale that fresh-ground aroma – your nose knows this is good food! Add a little kosher sea salt if you like.

Ground toasted Hempseed may be substituted for nuts, seeds, wheat germ, or bran. Alone or mixed with coffee it makes a tasty hot drink ("**Hava Narghila**," p. 57).

Refrigerate all Hempseed products: oil, flour or milk once opened, raw ground seed, toasted seed, and butter in tightly covered containers to maintain freshness. Use promptly. Freeze or refrigerate *dry* whole raw seeds; wet seeds will spoil in the refrigerator.

— As seen on Don't Tread on Me, 9/15/93
— Thanx to Ohio Hempery & to Lynn & Judy Osburn

Butter vs. Margarine

Dairy butter is not an ideal food, but is preferable to margarine in every way. Butter is especially useful for frying, baking, and heating because its saturated fatty acids are stable in high heat. Its short-chain fatty acids are easy to digest.

Margarine's unsaturated fatty acids, denatured in processing, are further destabilized by frying, creating indigestible free radicals. **Hempseed butter** and **oil** cannot be used for frying. etc., because they, too, are destabilized by high heat.

Recipe Abbreviations & Symbols

tsp. = teaspoon

T. = tablespoon

C. = cup

lb. = pound

(((= spicy

= medical cannabis recipe

= optional cannabis

Recipe Notes

_____

_____

_____

_____

_____

_____

_____

_____

_____

_____

_____

_____

_____

_____

Fixin's

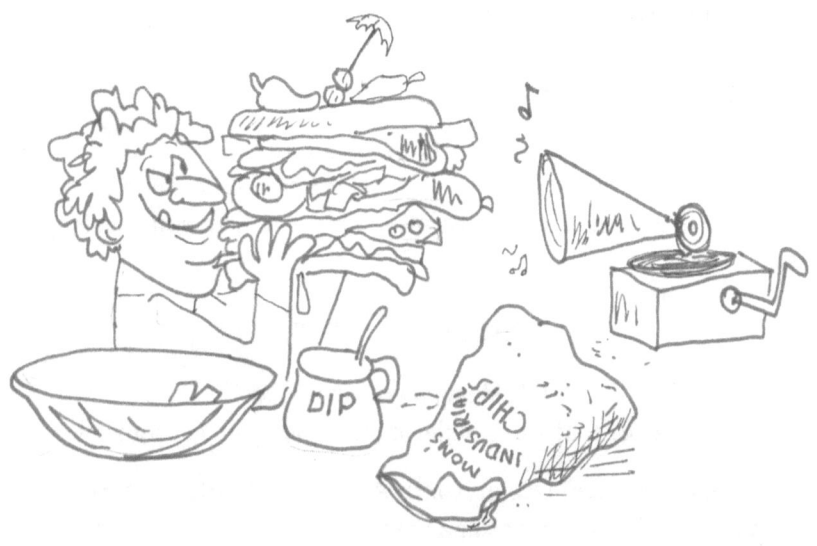

Using Hempseed Fixin's

Keep these items in the refrigerator for sandwiches, snacks, and other recipes included here.

Cinna-Hemp Toast Topping

For 4 pieces of toast, mix 2 T. sugar, 1 T. cinnamon, and 1/2 T. **ground toasted Hempseed** in a small container. Sprinkle on buttered slices of bread; toast in the oven or toaster oven.

Hempseed Breading

1 C. cornmeal, wheat germ, or seasoned bread crumbs
1/4 C. **ground toasted Hempseed**
1/2 tsp. salt
1/2 tsp. ground black pepper

Combine in a re-sealable bag to "shake'n'bake," "shake'n'fry," or oven-fry chicken, fish, okra (see **Kentucky Fried Okra**, p. 38), egg-coated zucchini rounds, or whatever you want to give a nice crispy crust.

Hempseed Tahini

1 C. **Hempseed butter**
1 T. sesame, sunflower, almond, safflower, or coconut oil

Blend until smooth. Use in North Asian and Middle Eastern foods as a substitute for sesame paste. See **Hempseed Tahini Salad**, p. 25.

— Adapted from the Hempseed Cookbook and used with permission.

"Hempricot" Marijuanade

1/2 C. honey   6 oz. apricot nectar
1/2 C. soy sauce   3 T. wok oil
3 T. crushed garlic   3 T. **raw ground Hempseed meal**
                    1 tsp. crushed red pepper flakes

Mix in a glass jar, cover tightly, refrigerate, and use to marinate tofu, beef, or chicken for stir fry. (See **"Sativory" Stir Fry**, p. 44.)

Savory Herbed Cream Cheese

8 oz. light cream cheese
2 T. minced chives
2 T. minced parsley

2 cloves minced garlic
2 T. minced basil
2 T. **ground toasted Hempseed**

1/3 C. Kalamata olives, pitted & chopped

Combine in a food processor, or by hand using a wooden spoon. Refrigerate. About an hour before serving, bring to room temperature. Serve with whole grain crackers, vegetable crudités, baguette rounds, or with sliced apples.

— *Adapted from the Hempseed Cookbook and used with permission.*

 see Twice-Baked Idaho POTato, p. 41

Spicy Hempseed Cheese

Mix 1 C. **hempnut** with water to moisten. Add two cloves chopped garlic, 1 tsp. red pepper flakes, 1 tsp. caraway or cumin seeds, and one packet (5 grams) kefir starter culture. Allow to ferment one day at room temperature. Pour through a filter paper or cheesecloth and refrigerate for 8 hours to stop fermentation and allow excess moisture to drain. Keep refrigerated; serve on bread or crackers.

— *Adapted from the Hempseed Cookbook and used with permission.*
— *Thanks to cheesemaker Christian of Austin Home Brew Supply for assisting this novice! — mgw*

Hempseed Caviar

A hempseed spread like this was eaten with flatbread in Finland in the 19th century. It will keep in the refrigerator for a week or so, but we can't keep it around that long!

Besides on flatbread, it's a great salad topping. And while the taste and aroma don't mimic fishy real caviar, it scores as high in essential fatty acids and looks like the real black variety!

1/2 C. whole raw hempseeds
1 T. olive oil
2 T. water
1/8 tsp. sea salt
1 tsp. dried or fresh lemon basil leaves, sage, or other herbs

Toast hempseeds in a deep, covered, dry frying pan, stirring constantly until seeds start "popping." Add other ingredients, and mix well with a hand-held electric mixer.

"Finnish Pizza"

On a piece of flatbread, layer sliced tomato and fresh mozzarella. Spoon 2 T. **Hempseed Caviar** on top. Place under broiler for 1 minute.

— Adapted from Goddess of Cake, http://goddessofcake.wordpress.com, and from a WASA® brand flatbread recipe insert.

Hempseed Oil Mayonnaise

Mayonnaise made with **Hempseed oil** is commercially available, or make your own:

In a blender, mix one egg, 2 T. white wine vinegar, 1 T. chopped fresh garlic, 1 tsp. mustard powder, salt and pepper to taste.

Slowly add 5 oz. fresh **Hempseed oil**. Continue to blend very slowly until proper consistency is reached.

Hemp Sandwich Spreads

Mix ingredients for your favorite in a blender or food processor. Invent your own using these as models. Cover and refrigerate for sandwiches or with soup & crackers.

For all varieties, start with
1 C. cooked mashed beans, lentils, or split peas
2 T. **Hempseed Oil Mayonnaise** (p. 18)

Oriental Wave (try with lentils)

2 C. hard tofu	1/2 C. dairy butter
1/2 C. ground toasted sesame seeds	Salt to taste
1/2 tsp. soy or tamari sauce	Chopped fresh garlic to taste

Italian Garden (try with Great Northern white beans)

2 T. grated Parmesan/Romano cheese	2 T. ricotta/cottage cheese
2 T. dairy butter	2 T. fresh finely chopped carrot
2 T. chopped onion	2 T. fresh finely chopped Bell pepper
1 T. chopped fresh garlic	1/2 tsp. dried/1 T. fresh chopped basil
1/2 tsp. dried/1 T. fresh chopped oregano	Salt to taste

Black pepper to taste

Sunshine Power (try with yellow split peas)
1/2 C. ground toasted sunflower, pumpkin, melon, or winter squash seeds
1/2 C. coarsely chopped peeled mango, Mandarin orange segments, and/or pineapple chunks

1/4 C. dairy butter	1/2 C. fresh finely chopped carrot
Salt to taste	Black pepper to taste

Hemp Dips

Mix 1/2 C. **Hempseed butter** into your favorite party dip and serve with chips and salsa. Some good combinations are hempseed bean dips, cheese dips, or guacamole.

For French onion dip, leave Hempseed butter slightly grainy, to complement the crunch of the onion.

Recipe Notes

_____

_____

_____

_____

_____

_____

_____

_____

_____

_____

_____

_____

_____

_____

_____

_____

_____

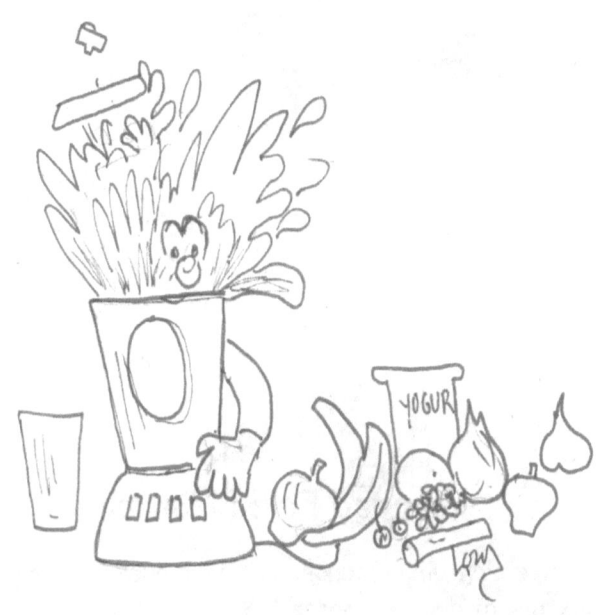

Fruits

Using Hempseed in Fruit Smoothies

Add 2 T. of **ground toasted** or **raw ground Hempseed** to any fruit smoothie and blend well for an added nutrient bounce! This is also a great way to use **hemp protein powder**!

Smoothies are a good vehicle for using medicinal cannabis leaves and flowers. Add to taste, according to your experience.

Hemp/Cayenne Mango Roll

Mix 1 T. **ground toasted Hempseed**, 1 T. ground cayenne pepper, and 1/2 T. salt. Peel and slice a ripe mango. Dredge pieces in Hemp/pepper mixture until well covered, then roll and secure with a toothpick.

Lights up your life! Spicy!

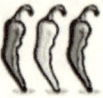

Hemped Fried Plantain

Slice a ripe plantain or banana for each guest into eighths and roll in a mixture of **ground toasted Hempseed** and wheat germ. Sauté pieces in dairy butter or coconut oil, turning frequently until browned on all sides. Drain on a paper towel. Great with rice and beans. For a light dessert, roll sautéed pieces in confectioner's sugar after draining!

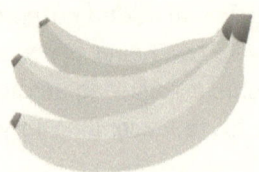

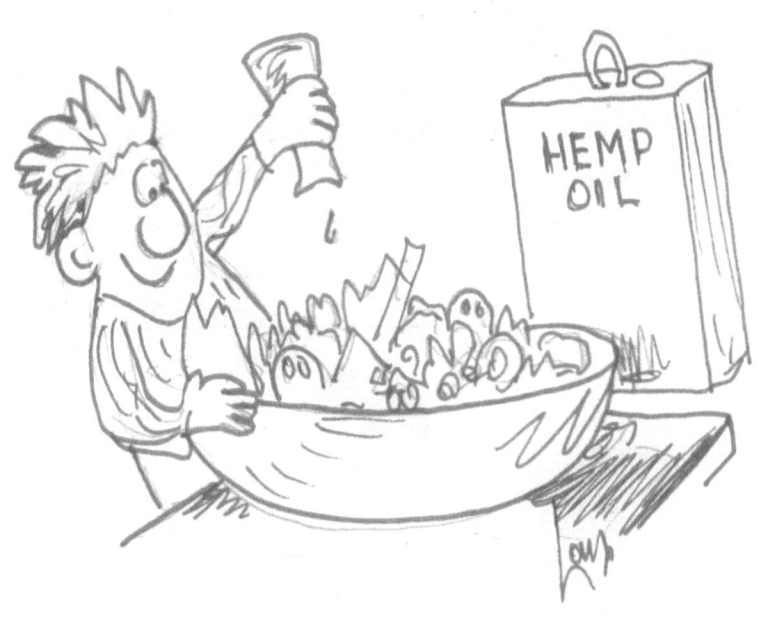

Salads & Salad Dressings

Using Hempseed in Salads & Salad Dressings

Hempseed is a crunchy, flavorful addition to any salad. Just sprinkle **ground toasted Hempseed** over the salad before serving, like croutons!

Or add 2 tsp. **raw ground Hempseed meal** to bottled or fresh salad dressings, shake well and savor!

Hempseed Salad Dressing

1 C. **Hempseed oil** or olive oil

1/2 C. sugar, honey, or substitute sweetener

1/2 C. wine vinegar

1 T. **raw ground Hempseed meal**

1 T. grated onion

1 tsp. dry mustard

1/2 C. red wine

1 tsp. salt

1/4-1/2 oz. ground marijuana or 1-3 g. flower tops *(optional)*

Put all ingredients except oil into a blender. Blend well on high speed, slowly adding oil. Chill. Serve with any green salad.

— Adapted from Brownie Mary's Marijuana Cookbook and Dennis Peron's Recipe for Social Change.

Hempseed Tamari Dressing

1/4 lb. hard tofu

1 T. **ground toasted Hempseed**

1 clove garlic, crushed

juice of one lemon, or 2 T. raspberry vinegar

1 C. fresh herbs (parsley, thyme, marjoram, &/or basil), chopped

1/2 small yellow onion, chopped

1/2 Bell pepper, chopped

1 T. tamari or soy sauce

1 C. **Hempseed oil** or olive oil

Put all ingredients except oil into a blender. Blend on high speed, slowly adding oil. Chill. Serve with any green salad.

— Adapted from the Hempseed Cookbook and used with permission.

Tabouley

1 1/2 C. **hempnut**

1/4 C. fresh mint, chopped

4-5 green onions, chopped

1/4 C. *pignolias* (pine nuts), coarsely chopped

1 bunch Italian parsley, chopped

2 Roma tomatoes, chopped

1 small cucumber, diced

2-3 T. olive oil

juice of 1 lemon

Mix all ingredients together. Best when chilled overnight.

— Adapted from Vegannosaurus Rex, http://vegannosaurus.com

Hempseed Tahini Salad
("Hempseed Hummus")

1 1/2 C. **hempnut**

2 tsp. salt

3 cloves garlic

2-3 T. olive oil

1 dried chipotle chile or other medium-hot red pepper

1/2-3/4 C. **Hemp Tahini** (see p. 16)

1/2 C. lemon juice (*or* brine from pickled hot peppers)

Dash of paprika

1/4 C. minced cilantro

(optional)

Put hempnut and salt in a saucepan with 2 C. water. Bring to a boil and simmer for ten minutes. Remove from heat and allow to cool slightly.

Grind or mince garlic cloves and chile in a food processor or blender. Add hempnut with its liquid, hemp tahini, lemon juice or pickle brine, and olive oil. Blend well and chill.

Turn the mixture out onto a shallow plate or platter. Pour another 2 T. olive oil over it. Use the back of a spoon to smooth and swirl the top. Dust with paprika and garnish with cilantro, if desired.

— Adapted from In Mol Araan, http://inmolaraan.blogspot.com

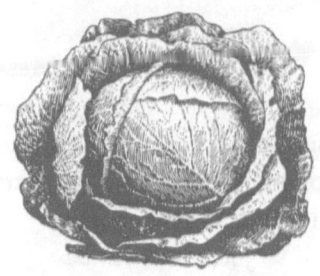

Stone Cole Slaw

1 head green cabbage, shredded   1 small red or white onion, diced
1 small head purple cabbage,   2 carrots, grated
   shredded
          1 small green Bell pepper, diced

Combine and mix all ingredients well in a large bowl.
Serve with:

Hemp Cole Slaw Dressing

1 C. **Hempseed Oil Mayonnaise** (see p. 18)
1 C. plain yogurt with active cultures
2 tsp. *comino* (cumin) seed, ground or whole (if whole, roll
the seeds briskly between your hands a few times to
release their flavor and aroma)
2 tsp. **ground toasted Hempseed**
1/2 C. apple cider vinegar
1/4 C. sugar, honey, *or* substitute sweetener

Mix well and pour over **Stone Cole Slaw**, folding dressing in
gently until vegetables are well covered. Chill for two hours and
serve. Great with barbeque and black beans, or with fried chicken
and potato salad!

Since 1975, Alaska has consistently allowed cannabis possession and cultivation for adult personal use despite ongoing challenges. We salute Alaska's vigilant Freedom Fighters with this delicious dish!

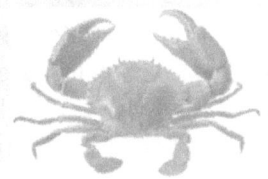

Alaska Stoned Crab Salad

1 pkg. rotini (corkscrew pasta), cooked according to directions & drained ("garden" varieties are pretty)
1 1/2 C. fresh spinach leaves, washed, drained & torn into pieces
1 1/2-2 C. fresh vegetables, chopped (any of these, or seasonal faves):

Bell pepper	onion	squash/zucchini
carrots	celery	cucumber
snap or sugar peas	tomato	broccoli or cauliflower flowerets

fresh Alaskan crabmeat in season, *or* 1 6-oz. can white crabmeat, drained
2 T. **ground toasted Hempseed**
3-4 T. **Hempseed Oil Mayonnaise** (see p. 18)
salt & pepper to taste
basil, thyme, rosemary *and/or* oregano to taste

Mix all ingredients gently in large salad bowl until crabmeat and mayo are fairly evenly distributed. Chill well. Serves 6-8.

Garnish with:
1 hard-boiled egg, crumbled; *and/or*
2 pieces of crisp bacon or 'bacon bits,' crumbled; *and/or*
1-2 dozen salad-size shrimp, boiled and peeled

— As seen on Don't Tread on Me, 10/20/93

Cozmic Chicken Salad

2 C. cooked chicken, chopped

1/2 C. **Hempseed Oil Mayonnaise** 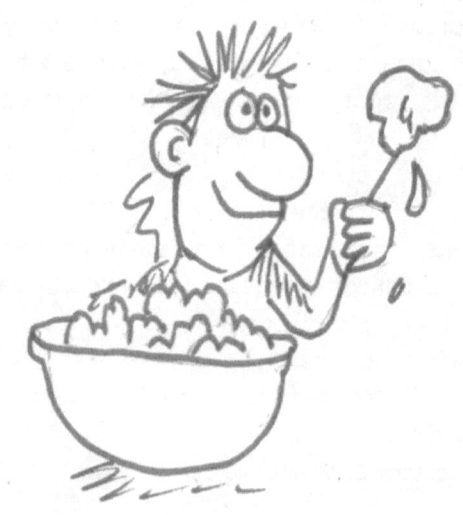(see p. 18)

1/2 C. onion, chopped

1/2 C. celery, chopped

1/2 C. apple, chopped

1/4 C. walnuts, chopped

1/8 C. Spanish olives, chopped

1 T. **ground toasted Hempseed**

Salt and pepper to taste.

Mix gently in large bowl until all ingredients are evenly distributed. Chill well. Serves 6.

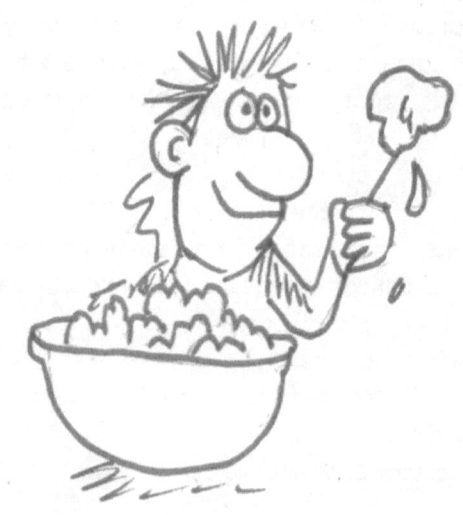

Soups

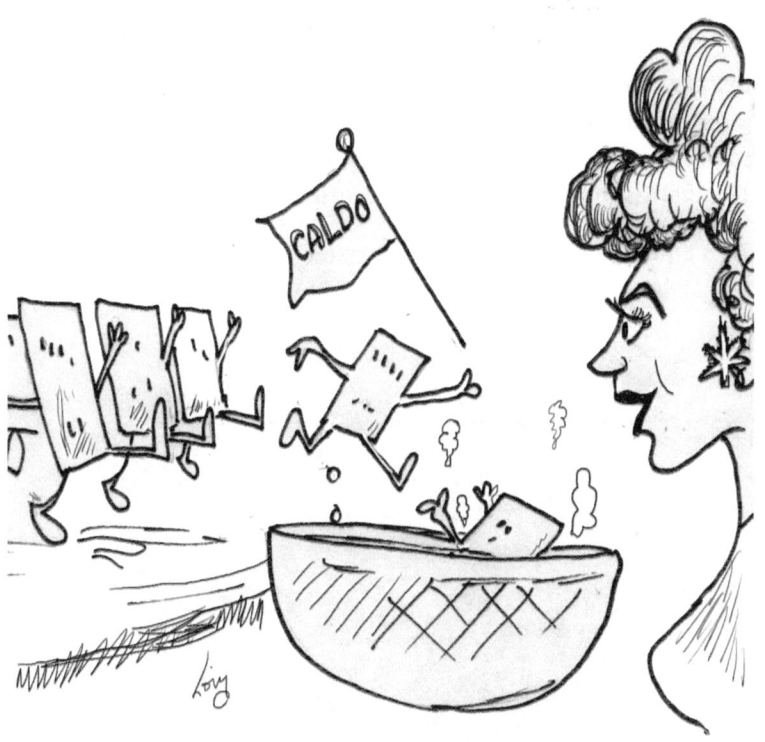

Using Hempseed in Soups

Make any soup or stew tastier by adding 2 T. to 1 C. ground toasted Hempseed.

Russian "Cannabage" Borscht

2 lbs. boneless soup meat, chopped   1 bunch beets, chopped
2 carrots, chopped   2 onions, chopped
3 stalks celery, chopped   1 Bell pepper, chopped
1 C. ground toasted Hempseed   1 tsp. salt
             2 T. sugar, honey, *or* substitute sweetener
                      12 oz. tomato paste
1 head cabbage, chopped   1 C. sour cream

Bring enough water to more than cover the meat to a boil in a large pot. Add meat and boil for 10 minutes. Add vegetables (except cabbage) and ground toasted Hempseed. Add salt and sweetener. Boil for 10 minutes; add tomato paste; continue boiling.

Add cabbage. Lower heat and simmer, covered, for 3 hours. Skim fat as it comes to the surface.

Serve hot with sour cream garnish. Serves 6.

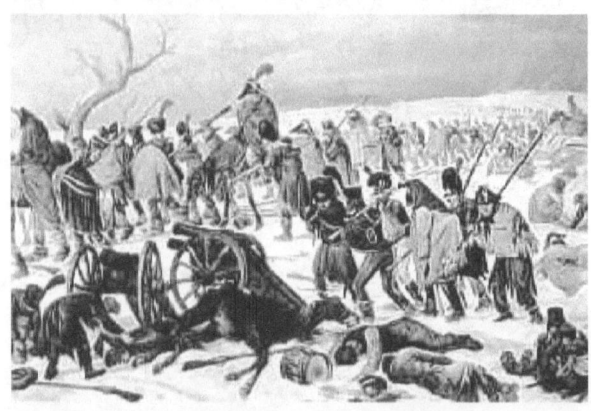

Russia has had prolific Hemp production for centuries, filling world demand for ships' canvas and rope. Russian peasants stayed alive through war and famine by eating Hempseed. The War of 1812 was fought in part to deny Napoleon Bonaparte's French empire control of Russian Hemp. With it, France could have ruled the seas and much of the world.

Indica Chill Soup

2 T. onion, chopped

2 T. dairy butter

2 T. curry powder

2 T. ground toasted Hempseed

1 T. flour

3 1/2 C. chicken or vegetable stock

4 egg yolks, slightly beaten

2 C. heavy cream

1/4 C. shrimp. cooked and peeled

In a large saucepan, sauté onion in butter until wilted. Add curry powder, ground toasted Hempseed, and flour and cook slowly for about 5 minutes. Pour in the stock slowly and bring to a boil, stirring. Reduce heat slightly. Add a few spoonfuls of this mixture to the egg yolks in a small bowl and stir well, then pour yolks into soup and simmer, stirring steadily, for a few moments. Don't let the soup come to a boil again!

Pour soup into a large serving bowl and chill thoroughly. Fold in cream. Ladle over shrimp in chilled soup bowls to serve 4.

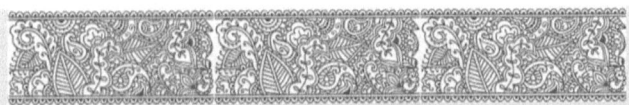

A Note on Curry

Curry powder has **curcumin**, the yellow pigment and active ingredient in turmeric (*Curcuma longa*). In India, where curry is consumed daily by virtually everyone, rates of cancer, diabetes, and cognitive disorders are considerably less than in the US and other Western countries. Curcumin and turmeric have strong anti-cancer, anti-cholesterol, anti-diabetic, antibacterial, antiviral, antifungal, and neuroprotective effects. They protect normal cells from the effects of chemotherapy and radiation, while increasing these treatments' effects on cancer cells. Curry powder includes other spices; plain turmeric is also widely available. Eat curry foods often! See **Hempseed Milk Curry Sauce**, p. 46.

Recipe Notes

_____

_____

_____

_____

_____

_____

_____

_____

_____

_____

_____

_____

_____

_____

Pasta Dishes

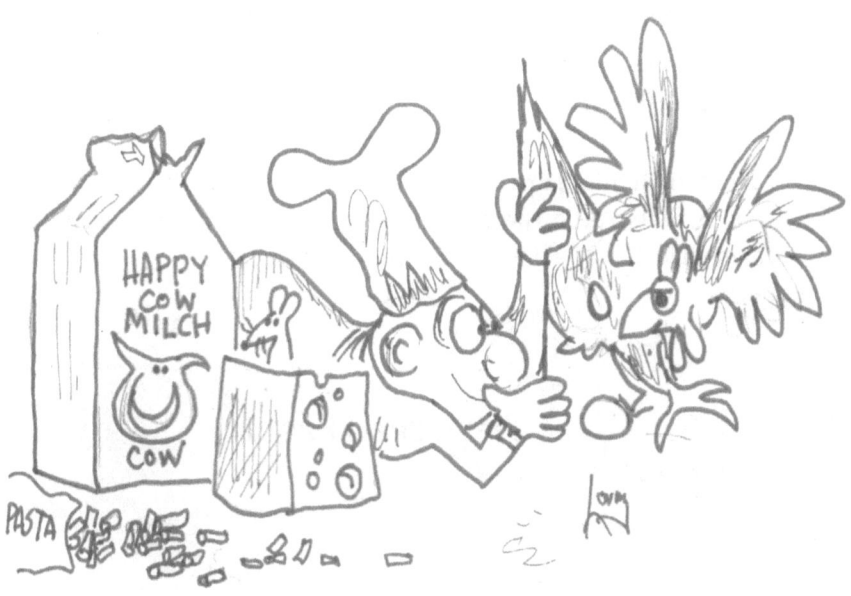

Hempseed Pasta

Commercially-made pasta with hempseed and other whole grains is available in many shapes and sizes. If you make your own pasta, you can easily incorporate **raw ground Hempseed meal**, **ground toasted Hempseed**, or **hempnut** into your recipes.

"Marijuanero" Sauce

3 T. olive oil
1 1/2 C. chopped onion
1 clove garlic, chopped fine
1 1-lb, 3-oz. can Italian plum
    tomatoes
1 6-oz. can tomato paste
1 1/2 C. water
salt and black pepper to taste
1/2 tsp. sugar, honey, *or* other
    sweetener
2 T. chopped cannabis leaves
    (optional)

1/2 tsp. dried *or* 2 sprigs fresh
    thyme
1 tsp. dried basil *or* 4 basil
    leaves, chopped fine
1 bay leaf
1 T. finely chopped parsley
1/4 C. **ground toasted Hempseed**

Cooked spaghetti or fettuccini

Heat oil in a large pot. Add onion and garlic. Cook on low heat until onion wilts. Add the other ingredients and simmer, stirring occasionally, for 30 minutes. Serve hot over pasta.

Hempseed Pesto

1 C. fresh basil
1/4 C. olive oil
2 cloves peeled, crushed garlic
1/4 C. **ground fresh Hempseed**
1/4 C. *pignolias* (pine nuts) *or* walnuts *(optional)*
1/2 tsp. sea salt
1/2 C. grated Parmesan cheese
2 T. **Hempseed butter** *or* dairy butter

Wash basil and remove stems. Pack tightly to measure. Combine with oil, garlic, ground Hempseed, nuts, and salt in food processor or blender and liquefy. Blend, briefly, with Parmesan cheese, and even more briefly with room-temperature butter.

Toss with hot cooked spaghetti or noodles. Serves 6.

— Thanks to Kate Braun, pasta chef extraordinaire!

Noodle Dairy-Hempseed Pudding

1 16-oz. package medium curly noodles
1 tsp. cinnamon
1/8 tsp. salt
1/2 C. raisins
1/2 C. chopped nuts (almonds or pecans)
1/4 C. **ground toasted Hempseed**
3/4 C. sugar, honey, or substitute sweetener
2 tsp. almond extract
2 C. dairy milk, **Hempseed milk**, or *prepared eggnog* (**extra rich!**)
3 eggs
1/4 lb. dairy butter

Prepare noodles as directed, rinse under cold water to remove excess starch and drain. Add cinnamon, salt, raisins, ground toasted Hempseed, sweetener, and almond flavoring. Mix together gently. Beat Hempseed milk, dairy milk, or eggnog together with eggs; add to noodles. Melt butter; add half to mixture.

Put remaining butter in a 9 x 12 baking dish, then pour in the noodle mixture. Bake at 350° until top is browned, about 25 minutes.

Allow to cool until pudding "sets." Cut into squares to serve 12. WARNING: this dish, especially if made with eggnog, is festively fattening; make it to share with 11 friends!

Recipe Notes

_____

_____

_____

_____

_____

_____

_____

_____

_____

_____

_____

_____

_____

_____

_____

_____

Vegetables

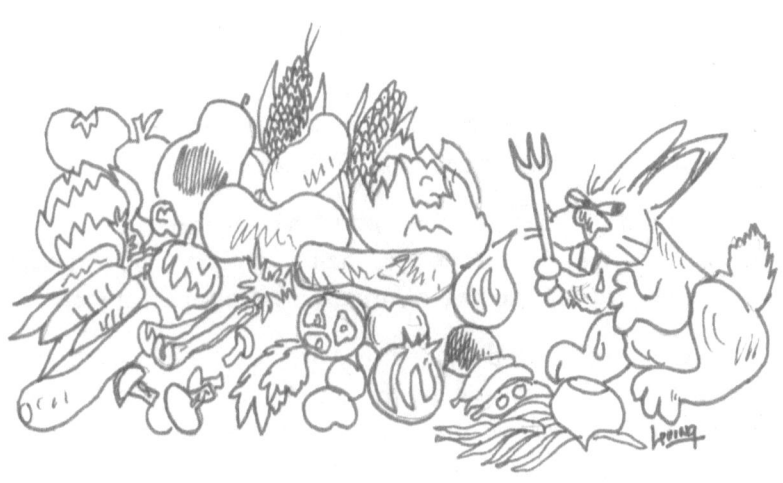

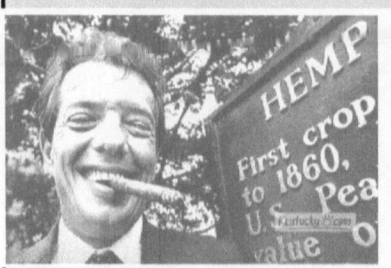

Kentucky was a premier Hemp growing state until Cannabis Prohibition. Parts of it uphold this tradition even in today's adverse legal climate! Five-time KY Gov. candidate Gatewood Galbraith (1947-2012) was a strong advocate for US Hemp and family farmers.

Kentucky Fried Okra

1 lb. fresh okra, cut into rounds
2 eggs, slightly beaten in a mid-
    size bowl
2 tsp. water

1 1/4 C. **Hempseed breading**
    (see p. 16)
corn, safflower, sunflower, or
    coconut oil for frying

Mix okra, eggs, and water in a bowl until okra is well moistened. Place **Hempseed breading** in a quart ziplock bag. Heat oil in a skillet until a drop of water will sizzle in it (or "oven-fry" — see below).

Using a slotted spoon, remove okra from egg mixture a spoonful at a time. Let excess egg drain off, then drop okra into the breading bag. Close bag tightly and shake until okra pieces are well-coated.

Remove okra from the bag (fingers are best), shake off excess breading gently, then place in hot oil and fry, turning gently until golden brown. Don't crowd the pieces. Keep the temperature just high enough that oil sizzles. Repeat until all okra is fried, removing from oil and draining on paper towels as they are done. Serve hot. Serves 4.

To Oven Fry:

Proceed as above, substituting other veggies if desired, or using chicken pieces, but do not heat oil in frying pan. Instead, heat oven to 400°. Remove coated okra or other food from breading bag and spread in a single layer on a baking sheet lightly coated with cooking oil. Bake until golden brown, turning once or twice.

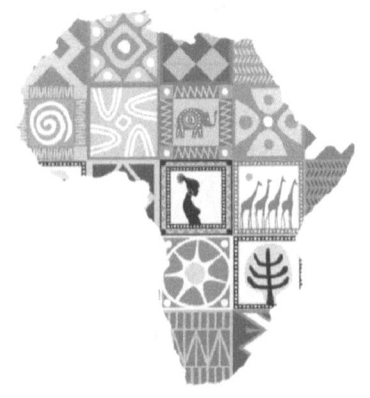

Squash, peppers, and Hempseed, from the plant families *Cucurbita*, *Capsicum*, and *Cannabis*, all were brought as precious hidden cargo to the Western Hemisphere by men and women kidnapped from Africa (though *Cannabis* had made the voyage long before). In the misery of the slave ships, they clung to Hope, Determination, and a few tiny Seeds, traveling to a future no one could have imagined.

The world today seems headed towards its own unimaginable fate - Re-Birth or Destruction, we cannot yet know. Do we have the Hope & Determination to be Seeds; to be Freedom Fighters?

Freedom Fighter Zucchini Hemp Casserole

1 medium zucchini per person, sliced in 1/8 inch rounds

for 3 - 5 zukes:

2 T. safflower or sunflower oil

salt and black pepper to taste

1/4 large onion, coarsely chopped

2 T. **ground toasted Hempseed**

salt, black pepper, basil, oregano, thyme and/or marjoram to taste

1/3 C. Italian-flavored bread crumbs

1 large tomato, *or* one can cooked, peeled, no-salt-added tomatoes, chopped

1/4 Bell pepper, diced

1 T. dairy butter

Put oil in ovenproof casserole dish. Cover bottom with a layer of sliced zucchini. Season lightly. Sprinkle chopped onion over zucchini. Add another layer of zukes and more seasoning. Cover with tomato pieces. Sprinkle **ground toasted Hempseed** and more herbs over tomato. Add a third layer of zucchini, season sparingly. Layer with Bell pepper pieces and more salt, pepper, and/or herbs.

Repeat until all ingredients are used. Cover and bake at 350° for 35-45 minutes (until zukes are tender). Remove cover, top with bread crumbs, dot with butter, increase heat to 375°, and bake 5 minutes more to brown. *Or* microwave for 25 minutes at a medium high setting. Omit bread crumbs and leave casserole covered unless you're using a microwave browning device.

Alternatives

1. For a main dish, add 1 C. cooked, chopped chicken to first layer, 1 C. fresh, frozen, or drained canned corn to second layer, and 2 chopped Serrano peppers to third layer. Spicy!

2. Substitute yellow or white squash for zucchini or use them mixed together.

3. Omit tomato. Add 1/2 C. shredded cheese to each layer (cheddar, mozzarella, and/or Colby are good).

— As seen on Don't Tread on Me, 9/22/93

Zucchini Hemp Seed Latkes

Latkes, usually made from potatoes, are traditionally enjoyed at the Jewish Passover – a Freedom celebration, not at all coincidental. Zucchini and hempseed are great together!

4 small zucchinis, 6-7" long
1/2 C. **whole raw hempseed**
4 T. fresh chopped dill weed,
   or 2 T. dried
1 1/2-2 1/2 C. chickpea flour + a bit more if needed (depends on size
   and juiciness of zukes)
salt
1/2 C. coconut milk
black pepper and/or
paprika to taste

1 C. grated Parmesan, Romano, and/or Asiago cheese
corn oil for frying

Grate zucchinis and place in a colander. Salt lightly and let drain for an hour. Soak hempseeds in water for the same length of time.

Drain hempseeds and grind in a food processor with coconut milk. Mix zucchini with hempseed, dill, about 1/2 tsp. more salt, and pepper/paprika if desired. Add chickpea flour and grated cheese. Mix well.

Heat oil to frying temperature in a large skillet. Spoon batter by Tablespoons into hot oil. Fry on both sides until golden. Drain on paper towels. Serve with rice and beans. Makes about 3 dozen.

*— Adapted from **In Mol Araan**, http://inmolaraan.blogspot.com*

Twice-Baked Idaho POTato

Bake a large potato until done. Allow to cool. Halve lengthwise and scoop out pulp, leaving potato skin "half-shells" intact.

Mix and mash potato with half again as much **Spicy Hempseed Cheese** or **Savory Herbed Cream Cheese** (p. 17), and 2 T. **ground toasted Hempseed**. *Optional:* add 2 T. fresh, chopped 🌿 cannabis flowers.

Spoon mixture back into potato skin shells, dot with dairy butter, and broil for 2 minutes or until top is golden brown.

Top with chopped chives, sour cream, and/or bacon bits. Serves one.

Crunchy Carrots

This dish is basically made by oven-frying (see p. 38), but uses no eggs and a slightly different technique:

4 large carrots, washed and lightly skinned
1 T. corn, sunflower, coconut, or safflower oil
1/2 C. **Hempseed Breading** (see p. 16)
Hempseed butter or dairy **butter**

Cut carrots into bite-size chunks. Brush lightly with oil. Put hempseed breading into a re-sealable bag. Add carrot chunks a few at a time, close bag tightly, and shake until pieces are well-coated.

Spread carrots one layer deep in an 11 x 14 inch baking dish and dot with butter. Cover tightly and bake at 350° for 30 minutes. Serves 4-6.

Yummy Yams

6 yams, a.k.a. sweet potatoes	1/4 lb. dairy butter
1/2 C. brown sugar	1/4 C. honey
1/8 C. hulled sunflower seeds	1/8 C. **ground toasted Hempseed**
dash of cinnamon	dash of ginger
⚡ 1/8 C. clean cannabis *(optional)*	tiny marshmallows *(optional)*

Boil yams for about 20 minutes. Cool, peel, and cut lengthwise. Place in an oven-proof dish. Preheat oven to 375°. Melt the butter and blend in a bowl with brown sugar and honey. Pour over potatoes. Add sunflower seeds, ground toasted Hempseed, and cannabis if desired. Sprinkle with ginger and cinnamon. Top with marshmallows if desired. Simmer, covered, in the oven for one hour. Serves 6 for a newly twisted Thanksgiving classic!

— *Adapted from The HiCentennial Marijuana Cookbook.*

Main Courses

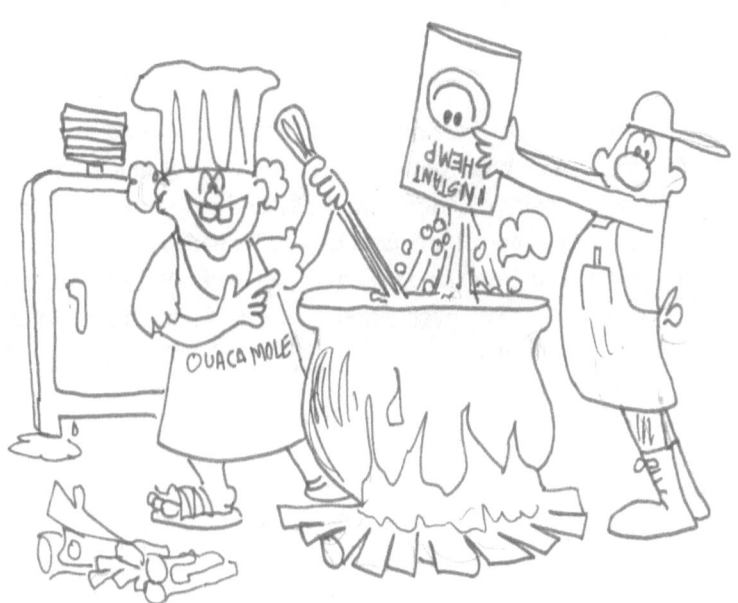

"Sativory" Stir Fry

For every 4 people:
8 oz. **"Hempricot" Marijuanade** (see p. 16)
1 box hard tofu, diced, *or* 1 lb. beef stew meat, cut thin
one chopped onion   one chopped Bell pepper
                                    wok oil
1 C. or more of each of three chopped or sliced vegetables, in season
                and to taste, *add more for more servings*:

cauliflower	broccoli
carrots	yellow squash, zucchini
baby bok choy	snow *or* sugar peas
Italian brown or Shiitake mushrooms	Mung bean *or* other sprouts

Marinate tofu or beef in **"Hempricot" Marijuanade** several hours or overnight in the refrigerator. Remove pieces to a bowl, conserving marinade.

Heat oil in a wok until sizzling. Add tofu or beef and stir-fry quickly. When tofu or beef begins to brown, push it aside and quickly add vegetables, cooking harder ones first and soft ones, such as snow peas, last. Add more marinade as you "wok" to prevent sticking. When everything has been added, cover, lower heat, and steam for one or two minutes. Serve over cooked rice or vermicelli noodles.

Chicken "Hempian"

3 whole chicken breasts
1 20-oz. can pineapple chunks
  (drain and reserve 3/4 C.
  juice)
1/2 C. dairy butter
1/4 C. **ground toasted Hempseed**

⚡ 1/4 C. clean, fresh
  marijuana, ground fine
  (optional)
1 T. cornstarch
3 T. lime juice
1 pkg. dry onion soup mix

Preheat oven to 350°. Split, bone, roll, and secure breasts with toothpicks. Arrange with pineapple in a 2-qt. baking dish. In a small pan, melt butter. Add ground toasted Hempseed, soup mix, and marijuana if using. Slowly add cornstarch, lime and pineapple juices. Pour over chicken. Bake 45 minutes. Test with a fork: chicken should be very tender. Serves 2.

— *Adapted from Cooking With Marijuana*

"Shremp" Banana Curry

2 lbs. large shrimp (shelled
  and de-veined)
1/3 C. + 2 T. dairy butter
1 medium onion, diced
6 T. flour
2 tsp. curry powder
1 1/2 tsp. sugar, honey, or
  substitute sweetener
1/4 tsp. ginger
1/2 C. **ground toasted Hempseed**

⚡ 1/3 C. clean, fresh
  marijuana, ground fine
  (optional)
2 C. dairy or **Hempseed milk**
1 C. chicken or vegetable
  bouillon
1/2 tsp. salt
1 tsp. lemon juice
4 medium bananas, sliced
  lengthwise

Hot cooked rice

Boil shrimp for 5 minutes and drain; set aside. In 1/3 C. butter in a saucepan, sauté onion until tender. Slowly blend in flour, curry powder, sweetener, ginger, and ground toasted Hempseed with a wire whisk. Add marijuana if desired. Add dairy or Hempseed milk and bouillon; stir constantly until curry thickens. Add salt and lemon juice. Add shrimp. Continue cooking until heated through.

Separately sauté bananas in 2 T. butter until lightly browned. Top hot rice with banana slices in 4 individual bowls. Pour curry and shrimp over all.

— Adapted from Cooking With Marijuana

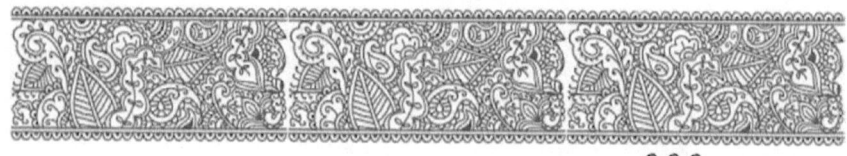

Hempseed Milk Curry Sauce

Sauté 1 T. minced garlic in a little oil until it starts to turn golden. Add about 1 tsp. ground black pepper, 1 tsp. cayenne pepper, 1/2 tsp. dried oregano, 1/2 tsp. dried rosemary, and a dash of thyme, sauté a little longer.

Add 1/2 C. **raw ground Hempseed meal** and 2T. curry powder. Reduce heat and continue cooking for about 2 minutes.

Slowly add 1 1/2 C. **Hempseed milk**. Stir constantly over low heat about 5 minutes, until sauce thickens. Serve over cooked rice and **Spicy Hempseed Pattie** (next page); or with grilled tofu, lamb, or chicken; or over peeled avocado halves. Serves 4.

— Courtesy One Love Caribbean Greille, Austin, TX

Spicy Hempseed Pattie (((

vegetable oil for frying
2/3 C. diced yellow onion
2 T. minced hot pepper
1/2 tsp. ground nutmeg
1/4 tsp. chili powder   1 15-oz. can pigeon peas or field peas, drained
2 T. peeled, minced ginger root   1 C. **raw ground Hempseed meal**
1/2 C. cooked rice   1 1/2 C. panko bread crumbs, divided
2 tsp. minced garlic
1/2 C. chopped button mushrooms
1 tsp. ground allspice
1/4 tsp. ground ginger
2 eggs, slightly beaten

Heat 2 T. oil in a skillet over medium heat. Add onions and garlic. Sauté for 2 minutes. Add mushrooms, sauté 3-4 minutes longer. As onions brown, add pepper and dry spices; sauté one minute more.

Using a slotted spoon, place the mixture into a large bowl and let cool slightly; wipe out skillet. In another bowl, mash peas lightly with a fork. Add peas, ginger root, raw ground Hempseed meal, rice, and half the panko crumbs to sautéed mixture. Add eggs. Mix well; will be somewhat sticky and chunky. Form into balls with wet hands, flatten. Dredge in remaining crumbs, pressing firmly into patties to coat.

Heat more oil and fry each pattie over medium high heat, 3-4 minutes on each side until browned and crisp; drain. *Or* stuff halved Bell peppers with mixture; bake 30 min. at 350°. Serve either version with **Hempseed Milk Curry Sauce** (previous page).

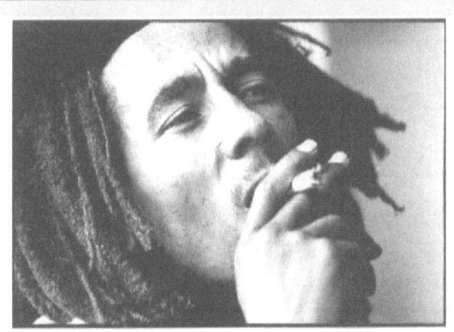

Jamaica
This spicy pattie evokes *ganja*'s amazing history in Jamaica, where Rastafarians consider cannabis a sacrament. Conscious reggae music, embodied in performers like Bob Marley (left), Peter Tosh, Jimmy Cliff, Sistah Carol, and hundreds more gives Freedom Fighters worldwide joy and strength to carry on. One Love!

Recipe Notes

_____

_____

_____

_____

_____

_____

_____

_____

_____

_____

_____

_____

_____

_____

_____

_____

Breads & Pastries

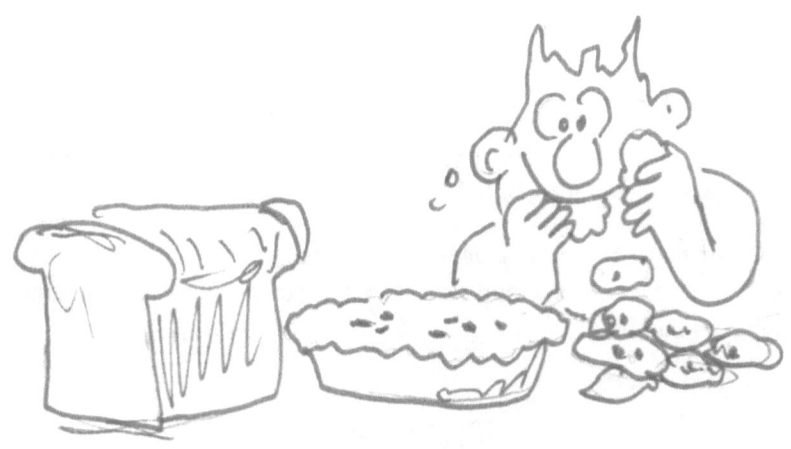

Add 1/2 – 1 C. **hempnut** to bread recipes – delicious!
See *Baking with Hempseed Meal*, p. 12, for more ideas!

Hemp Harvest Bread

4 eggs, beaten   2 C. sugar, honey, or other sweetener
2 C. canned, or cooked and mashed pumpkin   2/3 C. water
1 C. corn, sunflower, coconut, or safflower oil   1 3/4 C. wheat flour
1 3/4 C. white flour   1/2 tsp. baking powder
1 tsp. ginger   1 tsp. nutmeg
1 tsp. cinnamon   1 tsp. ground cloves
1/2 C. chopped nuts *(optional)*   1 C. raisins, or chopped dates or figs
1/2 C. **ground toasted Hempseed**

Add honey to eggs. Beat together. Add pumpkin, oil, and water; beat thoroughly.

Sift and mix dry ingredients. Add gradually to the pumpkin mixture. Blend well. Add nuts, ground toasted Hempseed, and dried fruit.

Fill four small greased loaf pans half full (the loaves rise). Bake at 350° F. for about 1 hour, until a toothpick inserted in the center of each loaf comes out clean.

Variations: Substitute overripe bananas; cooked, mashed sweet potatoes; or cooked, mashed acorn squash for pumpkin, or add any to pumpkin as you like.

Hemp Cornbread

1 C. flour   3/4 C. yellow cornmeal
1/3 C. sugar, honey, or substitute sweetener
3 tsp. baking powder   1/2 tsp. salt
1/2 C. **ground toasted Hempseed**   1 egg, well beaten
1 C. dairy milk or **Hempseed milk**
3 T. melted dairy butter or cooking oil

Preheat oven to 425° F. Grease an 8 x 8 inch baking pan or a muffin tin. Sift and mix dry ingredients. Add egg and milk, stir to mix. Add melted butter or oil and mix. Let rest for 3 or 4 minutes, then pour into pan. Fill pan or muffin cups halfway. Bake for 25 minutes or until golden brown.

Best Banana Bread

1 C. ripe bananas	3 tsp. lemon juice
2 eggs	1 C. brown sugar
1/2 C. **raw ground Hempseed meal**	1 1/2 C. flour
1/4 C. wheat germ	3 tsp. baking powder
3 tsp. baking soda	1/2 tsp. salt

1/2 C. clean, fresh marijuana, finely ground *(optional)*
1 C. chopped nuts (*optional*)

Preheat oven to 375° F. In a bowl, mash bananas with lemon juice until smooth. In another bowl, cream eggs, raw ground Hempseed meal, and sugar together. Add to bananas, stir well.

In a third bowl, mix remaining dry ingredients. Add to banana/egg mixture. Stir in nuts and/or cannabis if using.

The dough will be very stiff. Spoon into a greased loaf pan and bake for 35–45 minutes or until a toothpick inserted into the center comes out clean. Let cool before slicing.

— Adapted from Cooking With Marijuana

Hempseed-Enriched Pie Crust

Combine 1 C. pastry flour, 1/2 C. **ground toasted Hempseed**, and 1 tsp. salt. 'Cut in' 1/3 C. dairy butter with a knife and fork until dough consists of butter flakes coated with flour/hempseed mixture. Gradually add 1/4 C. cold water, working it in to the dough for a scant 30 seconds – the more you handle a pie crust, the less tender and flaky it will be!

Quickly roll out crust on a flour-covered surface to 1/4 inch thick. Lift gently into 8" pie pan. Center crust over pan before letting edges touch. Trim edge with a sharp knife and use a fork or fingers to press it down all the way around the pan.

Use for any single-crust pie or quiche. Try canned fruit fillings for easy cherry, berry, and other pies.

— Adapted from the Hempseed Cookbook and used with permission.

Lynn Osburn's Chocolate Chip Cookie Recipe

Grind 2 C. clean Hempseed to make **raw ground Hempseed meal**. Add 1/2 C. whole wheat flour and one tsp. baking soda.

Mix in a separate bowl: 1 C. honey, 1 egg, 1 tsp. vanilla extract and 1/2 tsp. salt. Add the Hempseed meal mixture and stir until blended. Add 1 or 2 T. plain yogurt and stir. Mix in 1 C. chocolate chips.

Place walnut-to-plum-sized drops of batter on a buttered cookie sheet. Bake at 325° F. for 15 minutes.

Hemp Power! Cookies

Delicious 'Go-Power' for kids of all ages!

1/2 C. dairy butter, softened	3/4 C. brown sugar
1 egg, beaten slightly	1 1/2 tsp. vanilla extract
1/2 tsp. salt	1/2 C. whole wheat *or* white flour
1/2 C. wheat germ	3/4 tsp. baking powder
1/2 C. **ground toasted Hempseed**	1 1/2 C. non-instant oatmeal
3/4 C. raisins	1/2 C. sunflower seeds or chopped nuts (*optional*)

Cream butter and brown sugar together. Add egg, vanilla, and salt. Beat well. In a separate bowl, mix together flour, baking powder, wheat germ, ground toasted Hempseed, and oats with a fork, then blend well with other ingredients. Add nuts & raisins.

Add 1 T. water if necessary so that cookies hold together. Form mixture into Tablespoon-sized balls. Place on a greased cookie sheet and bake for 10–12 minutes at 375° F.

— As seen on Don't Tread on Me, 10/6/93

THE Brownies

2 squares unsweetened baking chocolate

1/3 C. dairy butter	1 tsp. vanilla extract
1 C. sugar, honey, *or* substitute sweetener	2 eggs
3/4 C. sifted flour	1/2 tsp. baking powder
1/2 tsp. salt	1/2 C. chopped nuts

1/8 C. **ground toasted Hempseed**

1/8 C. clean cannabis leaves (*optional*)

Preheat oven to 350° F. and grease a square baking pan about 8 x 8 x 2 inches deep. Melt chocolate and butter together in a double boiler. Remove from heat and add vanilla. Beat in sweetener and eggs.

Measure the flour after sifting, then sift again with baking powder and salt. Stir in chocolate mixture. Add nuts and ground toasted Hempseed, and cannabis leaves if desired. Blend well.

Spread into pan and bake for 30–35 minutes. Cool and cut into squares. Makes 1 1/2 dozen brownies.

— Adapted from *The HiCentennial Marijuana Cookbook* and *Supermother's Cooking With Grass*

Hamantaschen are made during Purim, the Jewish Feast of Queen Esther. The triangle shape resembles the big hat of Haman, a royal advisor who plotted against Persia's Jews and was foiled by Esther's courage. Cream cheese or fruit fillings may be used, but Hamantaschen are often filled with poppy seeds.

Poppy seeds metabolize in the body to form the same compounds as heroin, opium, and morphine, and can give false positive results for opiates on drug tests. Fortunately, Hempseed doesn't present the same problem!

HamantascHempen

2 C. sifted flour   1 C. dairy butter

1/2 lb. plain cream cheese

Blend room temperature butter and cream cheese together well. Gradually add sifted flour. Make a ball of the dough. Wrap tightly with a clean damp cloth. Refrigerate overnight.

Roll out dough 1/8" thick on a well-floured surface. Cut in 3" squares and place 1 T. **Hemp Moan Filling** (below) in the center of each. Fold squares to make triangles. Pinch shut with wet fingers to seal. Bake on greased cookie sheet at 350° F. until golden brown (about 20 minutes).

The original poppy seed filling is called "Mohn filling," but this version will make you *moan* with delight!

Hemp Moan Filling

1/2 C. **ground toasted Hempseed**   1 C. walnuts, chopped fine
1 C. golden raisins, chopped fine   honey

Combine ground toasted Hempseed, nuts, and raisins with enough honey to bind the mixture together.

Choco-Mondo Hempseed Torte

3/4 C. dairy butter

1/2 C. honey

1 3/4 C. ground almonds

6 eggs, separated

1 C. chocolate chips, melted

1/2-3/4 C. **ground toasted Hempseed**

Whip butter vigorously. Beat in egg yolks one at a time. Beat in honey. Mix in melted chocolate chips, almonds, and ground toasted Hempseed.

Beat egg whites in a separate bowl until stiff, and fold gently in to the Hempseed-almond mixture.

Bake in two 8" or 9" round cake pans at 375° F. for 10 minutes. Lower heat to 325° and continue baking for 20 minutes. Allow to cool completely before turning layers out one at a time onto a serving platter. Frost top of bottom layer with **Chocolate Chip Frosting**, below; stack second layer on it; then frost top and sides of torte.

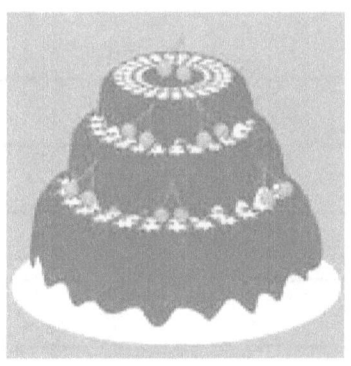

Chocolate Chip Frosting

1 C. chocolate chips

6 T. cream

1 T. butter

Melt chips and butter together. Add cream. Stir well.

— Reprinted with permission from the Hempseed Cookbook.

Recipe Notes

Breakfast

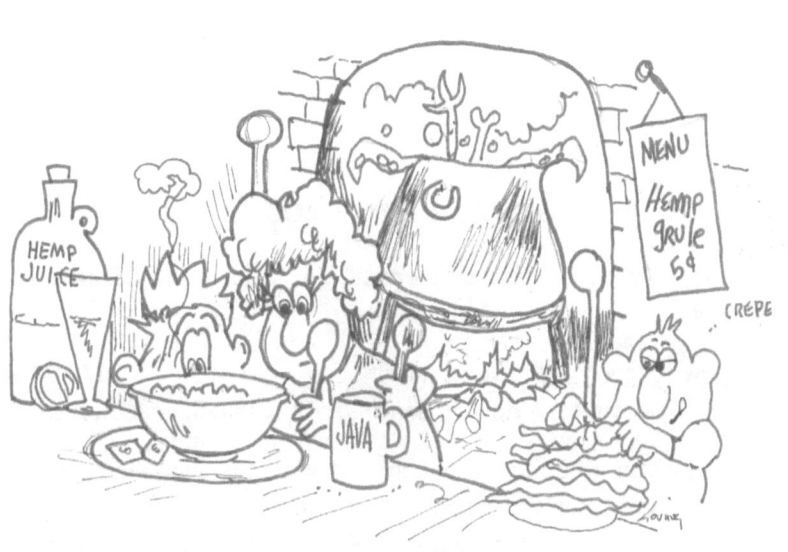

"Hava Narghila"
(A Hot Hemp Drink)

Doubling your usual coffee measure, substitute **dark toasted ground Hempseed** for all or part of coffee in any drip coffeemaker. Sweeten or cream to your taste, or drink 'black.' Made with Hempseed alone, caffeine-free Hava is like mild green tea — coffee fiends may initially find it pale, but grow to love it.

Himalayan Highland Lhassi

1 C. plain soy yogurt
1/4 C. **hempnut**
2 tsp. brown rice syrup or maple syrup

1 ripe banana, sliced
1 T. rose water (found in
Middle Eastern markets)
pinch ground cardamom

Place all ingredients in blender. Puree until smooth. Serve at room temperature or slightly chilled.

— *From the HempNut Cookbook*

Twisted Hempseed Gruel

Oliver's gruel — "More, please!" You'll love the Dickens out of this one!

1/4 C. **raw ground Hempseed meal**   1/2 C. water
  1/4 C. Cream of Wheat®, non-instant oatmeal, or Wheatena®

Bring water to boil in a saucepan. Add raw ground Hempseed meal, lower heat, and cook for 5 minutes. Add Cream of Wheat, oatmeal or Wheatena, stir well, cover and cook 5 more minutes. Remove from heat and let stand, covered, until desired consistency is reached.

Sweeten with honey, maple syrup, or brown sugar, and serve with cold dairy milk, **Hempseed milk**, or apple juice, and seasonal fruit or berries. One serving.

— *Adapted from the Hempseed Cookbook and used with permission.*

In addition to **Twisted Hempseed Gruel**, many commercially-prepared cereals contain varying amounts of hempnut or hulled hempseed. Granola and energy bars can also be found with healthy hempseed inside!

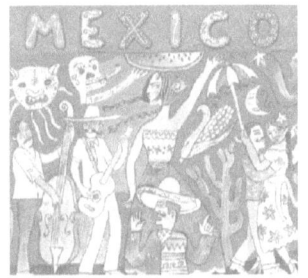

Mexico's "illegal" Cannabis growers, against intense government attack (including aerial spraying with US-provided poisons), sustained generations of US users. Not least among reasons to end the drug war is to relieve the people of Mexico of unparalleled state and criminal violence in turf wars over a valuable plant that could boost the Mexican economy and halt the exodus of Mexicanos to other nations.

Quiche Migas ofrece un saludo a nuestros amigos al otro lado dela frontera. ¡Vayan bien, hasta la victoria!

Quiche Migas

6 eggs, lightly beaten	1/2 C. milk

2 C. shredded cheese (cheddar, Monterey jack, or Colby)

2 T. dairy butter

2 large tomatoes, wedged	1/2 medium onion, diced
1/2 Bell pepper, diced	6 Italian mushrooms, sliced

3 Serrano or jalapeño peppers, chopped fine

2 C. corn tortilla chips, lightly crushed	1/4 C. **ground toasted Hempseed**

Combine eggs, milk and cheese in a bowl. In a skillet, sauté vegetables in butter. Add tortilla chips and ground toasted Hempseed when veggies are just tender; cook for only a minute or so longer. Remove from heat. Add sautéed veggies to eggs.

Pour into prepared **Hempseed-Enriched Pie Crust** (see p. 51) or a plain pastry crust. Bake at 350° F. until lightly browned and firm (15-20 minutes). Serve with *salsa* on the side.

Or pour egg mixture over sautéed vegetables in skillet and "scramble" to desired firmness, adding chips and Hempseed when nearly done. Serves 4 either way. Spicy!

Spiced Apple-Hemp Muffins

1/2 C. whole wheat pastry flour, sifted
1 C. ground oatmeal (puree in food processor to flour-like consistency)

1 C. **raw ground Hempseed meal**	1 tsp. cinnamon
3 tsp. baking powder	1 C. unsweetened applesauce
1/4 tsp. salt	1/2 C. maple syrup or agave nectar
1/2 tsp. ground nutmeg	3/4 C. dairy or **Hempseed milk**
1/4 tsp. ground cardamom or	1 tsp. vanilla extract
allspice	3 T. olive oil

Preheat oven to 350° F. In large bowl, combine all dry ingredients. In another bowl, combine all wet ingredients. Combine both together until just blended. Fill baking cups or greased muffin tins half-way with batter. Bake 30 min. for regular or 21-22 min. for mini-muffins, until a toothpick inserted in the center comes out clean. Makes 2 dozen regular or 48 mini-muffins.

Roll One Crepes

1/2 C. all-purpose flour	1/2 C. **Hempseed flour**
1 tsp. cornstarch	2 C. dairy or **Hempseed milk**
1/8 tsp. salt	2 eggs
1 additional egg yolk	1/4 C. dairy butter, melted

Place dry ingredients in a bowl. Mix well. Add eggs and milk; whisk until smooth. Add butter, whisk until well mixed. Refrigerate for about 30 minutes.

Heat a medium size non-stick pan or griddle on medium heat. Take batter from refrigerator, whisk again. Pour about 2 oz. at a time onto hot pan. Cook on one side 1 1/2 minutes, flip gently with a spatula, cook one more minute. Set aside until all are cooked.

Fill with scrambled eggs, jelly, bacon, ice cream; roll them in confectioner's sugar, cover with syrup, or not – find your favorites and enjoy them all!

— *Adapted from http://www.Hempseed.com*

A Few Representative Links & Resources, from among 1000s

General Cannabis/Hemp Information

JackHerer.com. www.jackherer.com * Keeping the work and memory of the man who kept hemp alive evergreen.

Cannabis Resource. www.cannabisresource.com * Independent info, answers, links, tweets, more.

Hemp Industries Association (HIA). http://thehia.org * Represents the hemp industry in Washington DC and states; encourages R&D on new products from industrial, low-THC oilseed, and fiber varieties of *Cannabis*.

Whole Hempseed & Hempseed Foods

Chi Hemp Industries. www.Hempseed.ca * Canada's premier source for hempseed, hempseed oil, and hemp foods.

Happy Hemp. hwww.happy-hemp.com * Minimally processed, super-fresh hempseed.

Manitoba Harvest. www,manitobaharvest.com * World's largest vertically-integrated hempfoods maker. More recipes on their website!

My Parrot Food.com. www.myparrotfood.com * Free shipping, low prices.

Nutiva. www.nutiva.com * Founded on hempseed oil, Nutiva now offers a variety of seeds and seed oils.

Nuts.com. www.nuts.com * Low prices, fast service.

Spice Sage Worldwide. www.myspicesage.com * Canadian bulk hempseed.

Cannabis Medicine

American Botanical Council. www.herbalgram.org. * Providing science-based and traditional information to promote responsible use of herbal medicines.

Americans for Safe Access (ASA). www.safeaccessnow.org * The largest US organization of patients, medical professionals, scientists, and citizens promoting safe, legal access to cannabis.

Cannabis International Foundation. www.cannabisinternational.org * Researching medicinal benefits of dietary cannabis, especially the fresh green leaves.

O'Shaughnessey's. www.beyondthc.com * *The journal of cannabis in clinical practice.*

Patients Out of Time. www.medicalcannabis.com * Patient advocates educate healthcare providers and policymakers about medical cannabis.

Advocacy Groups

Vote Hemp. www.votehemp.com * Dedicated to changing the law to allow US farmers to grow industrial, low-THC oilseed, and fiber varieties of *Cannabis*.

National Organization for the Reform of Marijuana Laws (NORML). www.norml.org * US' leading activist network, with chapters everywhere.

Cannabis Information Network. www.cinllc.org * Advocacy training, education, support.

Citizens Opposing Prohibition (COP). www.citizensopposingprohibition.org * Effective lobbying by former cops, prosecutors and just plain folks, making a difference in DC.

Harm Reduction Coalition. http://harmreduction.org * Advancing harm reduction policies, practices, and programs to address adverse effects of drug use including overdose, HIV, hepatitis C, addiction, and incarceration.

Marijuana Policy Project (MPP). www.mpp.org * Supporting change at state and federal levels. Monitors marijuana-related legislation in all 50 states.

Students for Sensible Drug Policy (SSDP). www.ssdp.org * Future leaders opposing the drug war now, planning and working for change they want to see.

Drug War History, News, & Discussion

420 Magazine. www.420magazine.com * Free membership gives access to news, online forums.

Cannabis News. www.cannabisnews.com * Constant news and policy updates.

Cannabis Network Radio. www.cannetradio.com * Live shows Tues & Thurs with host David Kowalsky. Streaming 24/7 with insider news, celebrity interviews and more.

Cannabis Now Magazine. www.cannabisnowmagazine.com * News, reviews, analysis.

Celeb Stoner.com. www.celebstoner.com * Hip and happening news highlights cannabis culture in all its many forms.

DRCNet Foundation/Stop The Drug War. www.stopthedrugwar.org * Publishes the online *Drug War Chronicle*, with comprehensive coverage of the war on drugs since 1997.

Drug Sense/Media Awareness Project. mapinc.org * A worldwide network dedicated to drug policy reform. Constant news updates.

High Times Magazine. www.hightimes.com * *Essential* cannabis news, views, and advocacy since 1974. High Times' Chef Ra was a pioneer in culinary cannabis use; kudos! Also see *High Times Medical*, www.hightimes.com/read/high-times-medical-marijuana.

Time 4 Hemp Radio. www.time4hemp.com * LIVE shows every Mon - Fri at 10-11 am PST. Archives.

Truth: The Anti-Drug War. www.briancbennett.com * Independently maintained cache of official government data and historic news reports document the war on drugs.

Weed World Magazine. www.weedworld.co.uk * Brit publication stresses healthy use and medical user information.

Bibliography

—. Marijuana prosecutions for 2010 near record high. Sept. 19, 2011. www.norml.org/news/2011/09/19/marijuana-prosecutions-for-2010-near-record-high.

Anonymous. **Supermother's Cooking With Grass.** Sunshine Mfg. & Import Co./Flash Mail Order Post Express Co., San Rafael, CA. 1971.

Armentaro P. **Emerging Clinical Applications for Cannabis and Cannabinoids.** NORML Foundation. Washington, DC. 2010. See at: www.norml.org

Callaway JC, Schwab U, Harvimaa I, et. al. Efficacy of dietary hempseed oil in patients with atopic dermatitis. *Journal of Dermatological Treatment.* 2005;16:87-94.

Camille CJ. **The HiCentennial Marijuana Cookbook.** Realtoys, Minneapolis, MN. 1976.

Erasmus U. **Fats and Oils.** Alive Books, Burnaby BC, Canada, 1986.

Flowers T. **the marijuana herbal cookbook..** Flowers Publ., Berkeley, CA. 1995.

Goddess of Cake. http://goddessofcake.wordpress.com.

Hemp Canada. http://www.Hempseed.caH.

Hemp Oil Canada, Inc., Shaun Crew, President. Laboratory Analysis of THC Content in Industrial Hemp Seed. Mar. 10, 2000.

Herer J. **The Emperor Wears No Clothes,** 11th ed.. Help End Marijuana Prohibition Van Nuys, CA & AH HA Publ., Austin, TX. 1998, 2000.

Holland J, ed. **The Pot Book..** Park Street Press, Toronto, CAN. 2010.

In Mol Araan. http://inmolaraan.blogspot.com.

Johnson R.. Hemp as an agricultural commodity. *Congressional Research Service.* Mar. 21, 2013.

Jones I. **The Grub Bag.** Vintage, NYC, 1971.

Lee MA. **Smoke Signals.** Scribner, NYC. 2012.

Miller C, Wirtshafter D. **Hempseed Cookbook..** Ohio Hempery, Athens, OH. 2001.

Osburn L. Hemp seed: the most nutritionally complete food source in the world. *Hemp Line Journal,* July-Aug. 1992; I(1):14-15.

Rathbun M, Peron D. **Brownie Mary's Marijuana Cookbook and Dennis Peron's Recipe for Social Change.** Trail of Smoke Publ., San Francisco, CA. 1993.

Restak RM. **Receptors.** Bantam Books, NYC. 1994.

Rezapour-Firouzi S, Arefhosseini SR, Farhoudi M, et. al. Association of Expanded Disability Status Scale and cytokines after intervention with co-supplemented hemp seed, evening primrose oils and hot-natured diet in multiple sclerosis patients. *Bioiimpacts.* 2013;3(1):43-47. http://www.ncbi.nlm.nih.gov/pmc/articles/PMC3648912.

Rose R. Hempseed foods. http://www.hempfood.com

Rose R, Mars B. **HempNut Cookbook..** The Book Publishing Co., Summertown, TN. 2004.

Rosenthal E, Gieringer D, Mikuriya T. **The Medical Marijuana Handbook..** Quick American Archives, Oakland, CA. 1997.

Russo E. History of *Cannabis* and its preparations in saga, science, and sobriquet. *Chemistry & Biodiversity.* 2007;4:1614-1648.

Russo EB, Grotenhermen F, eds. **Handbook of Cannabis Therapeutics.** The Haworth Press; New York, London, Oxford. 2006.

Schmevelyn E. **Cooking with Marijuana.** Sun Magic Publ., Seattle, WA. 1974.

Vegannosaurus Rex. http://vegannosaurus.com

Zimmer L, Morgan JP. **Marijuana Myths, Marijuana Facts.** The Lindesmith Center; NYC, San Francisco, CA. 1997.

Amino Acid Profile

AMINO ACID	Per 30g Serving
ALANINE	540mg
ARGININE	1494mg
ASPARTIC ACID	1240mg
CYSTINE	204mg
GLUTAMIC ACID	2097mg
GLYCINE	546mg
HISTIDINE	342mg
ISOLEUCINE	492mg
LEUCINE	828mg
LYSINE	486mg
METHIONINE	276mg
PHENYLALANINE	552mg
PROLINE	510mg
SERINE	612mg
THREONINE	417mg
TRYPTOPHAN	147mg
TYROSINE	387mg
VALINE	609mg

Essential Amino Acids

Hempseed's Amino Acids

Figure 5.

Index

70

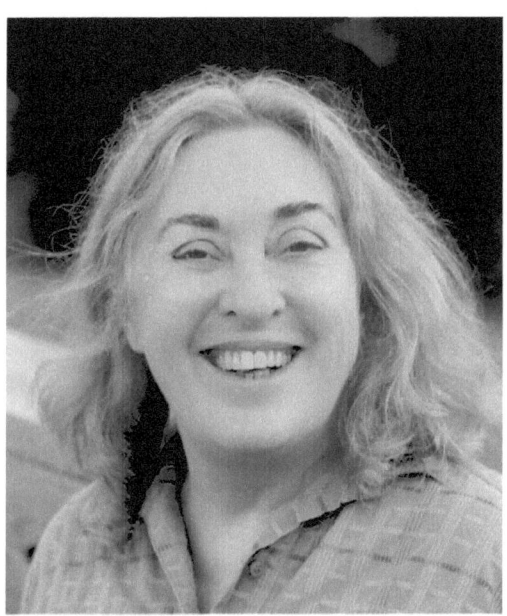

photo by Alan Pogue http://www.documentaryphotographs.com

Mariann Garner-Wizard is an Austin-based freelance writer, editor, and activist. A founder of the Texas Hemp Campaign, she has researched and written about harms of Cannabis Prohibition such as paraquat spraying and the losses of civil liberties, judicial independence, and environmentally safe Hemp fiber and fuel since the 1970s. When she began to learn about the lost nutrition of Hempseed, the seed for this book was planted.

Garner-Wizard writes regularly for HerbClip®, a peer-reviewed service of the American Botanical Council, evaluating medical cannabis studies among other topics. She reports on cannabis matters for ABC's quarterly journal, *HerbalGram*, and her incisive analysis has appeared in the *Bulletin of Cannabis Reform*. She hosts CannabisResource.com, an independent website with links, information, and organizer tools. She is a Contributing Editor of *The Rag Blog*, www.theragblog.blogspot.com.

Today, researchers are re-discovering the benefits of hempseed foods. Sooner or later, connections between hempseed's essential fats and amino acids, human endocannabinoid and nervous systems, and the nutritional causes of many chronic diseases (steadily rising in prevalence since Cannabis/Hemp Prohibition began) seem certain to emerge.

You are what you eat. As Grace Slick sang in *White Rabbit*, "Feed your head! Feed your head! Feed your head!"

www.ingramcontent.com/pod-product-compliance
Lightning Source LLC
Chambersburg PA
CBHW022338290526
45785CB00017B/2060